THIS IS A SOUL

THIS IS A SOUL

The Mission of Rick Hodes

M ARILYN B ERGER

WILLIAM MORROW
An Imprint of HarperCollins*Publishers*

Grateful acknowledgment is made to the following for the use of the photographs that appear throughout the text: collection of the author (pp. 137, 160, 180, 184, 187, 206, 242, 256, 257, 259); courtesy of Rick Hodes (pp. 6, 143); courtesy of Chloe Malle (pp. 13, 110, 140, 157, 158, 198, 224); courtesy of the American Jewish Joint Distribution Committee (pp. 53, 56, 80 top, 80 middle, 80 bottom, 81 top, 81 bottom); courtesy of Amit Desai (p. 68); photograph by JoAnn Silverstein (pp. 141, 150 bottom, 151 top, 151 bottom); photograph by Samantha Reinders (pp. 150 top, 175, 176, 190, 195); photograph by Danny Hodes (p. 222).

HarperCollins books may be purchased for educational, business, or sales promotional use. For information please write: Special Markets Department, HarperCollins Publishers, 10 East 53rd Street, New York, NY 10022.

FIRST EDITION

Designed by Jamie Lynn Kerner

Library of Congress Cataloging-in-Publication Data

Berger, Marilyn, 1950–
    This is a soul : the mission of Rick Hodes / Marilyn Berger.—1st ed.
    p. cm.
    ISBN 978-0-06-175954-3
    1. Hodes, Richard. 2. Physicians—United States—Biography.
3. Missionaries, Medical—Ethiopia—Biography. 4. Missions,
Medical—Ethiopia.
    I. Title.
    R722.32.H63B47 2010
    610.92—dc22
    [B]
                                 2009051271

10 11 12 13 14   OV/RRD   10 9 8 7 6 5 4 3 2 1

For Don,
who made magic with four words,
Tell Me a Story

And for Danny,
who became part of this one

You can be kind and true and fair and generous and just, and even merciful, occasionally. But to be that thing time after time, you have to really have courage.
　　　　　—Maya Angelou, Convocation Address,
　　　　　　　　　Cornell University, May 24, 2008

CONTENTS

Contents

THIS IS A SOUL

THIS IS A SOUL

HE WAS THE MOST BEAUTIFUL CHILD I had ever seen—and certainly the dirtiest. I came upon him in the middle of a crowded
sidewalk, crouched in front of the Florida Pastry, a small bakery
on Arat Kilo, one of the main avenues of Addis Ababa. Hundreds of pedestrians, from his vantage point probably a forest of
legs and sandaled feet, were gliding by in that distinctive and ele-
gant walk typical of Ethiopians. A row of shoeshine boys waited
for customers; a few peddlers hawked toothbrushes and shoes
and jeans and shirts.

The small boy looked to me to be about four years old, his
tiny right hand cupped skyward to catch the occasional coin that
came his way, his eyes staring up at me through impossibly long
and dusty eyelashes. His arms were no bigger around than a
garden hose, and his filthy green T-shirt outlined a back that was

humped out in a perfect pyramid. I'd been in the Ethiopian capital of Addis Ababa for just a few days, but I had already learned
that this was a sure sign of tuberculosis of the spine.

I happened to be walking on this particular day instead of
taking my customary $1.50 taxi ride, enjoying a moment to relax
because I'd completed all my reporting and was satisfied I'd
gotten the story I came for. I was returning to my hotel from the
clinic where Rick Hodes, an American doctor, treats impoverished children who have any number of diseases, the worst being
TB of the spine, scoliosis, heart disease, and cancer. He takes on
the most intractable cases, particularly when there is a chance of
a cure. I had come here to write about Dr. Hodes, not only because he has devoted his life to ministering to some of the poorest
people on the planet, curing what he can, ameliorating what he
cannot. That is rare enough for this product of America's sub-
urbs. What had particularly grasped my imagination was the
way he lives in this impoverished country. He has taken some
twenty poor and sick children into his own house and officially
adopted five of them. He cares for them, feeds them, and sends
every one of them to private school.

When I started to reach for some money to put into the outstretched hand of the small boy in the street, I remembered that
I'd been told it's wrong to give money to beggars, that the right
thing to do is to support organizations that help them.

There are hundreds, even thousands of children begging in
the streets of Addis, or so I thought. I was wrong by a long shot.
UNICEF reported in 2007 that there are five million orphans in
Ethiopia, one of the largest populations of orphans in the world,
and the number has been steadily increasing as more and more

children are orphaned by AIDS. With no other means of support, these children end up looking for handouts on the street.

Still, of all the beggars in Addis, I was haunted by the one little fellow with the deformed back. I kept replaying in my mind the way he looked directly at me with his gorgeous pleading eyes, and I couldn't wait to tell Rick about the boy who had the precise disease that he could cure.

An hour later, I was in Rick's clinic, which sits outside the chapel of the Mother Teresa home for the destitute in Addis, where the Missionaries of Charity carry on the work of their renowned founder. The sisters, all identically dressed in their blue-trimmed white linen saris, cheerfully minister to some six hundred sick and dying men, women, and children. They oversee an enclave of neat dormitories nestled behind a blue metal gate guarded by a genial but firm man who has to have the fortitude to turn away even more of the sick and dying. As desperate as the condition of the people inside the gate may be, those clustered outside are the street people with no shelter or care at all.

A neat border garden greets those who make it inside, and off to the left is the chapel and a small room set aside for Rick's clinic, furnished only by a table and a few chairs and totally devoid of any medical equipment. Patients hoping to see him line up outside where they can sit on a low stone wall. Kids from the mission hang around on the days Rick is there, some hoping to be invited out for a glass of juice when he takes a break.

About a dozen years ago, Rick started volunteering at the mission in what he liked to call his "free time." But that soon became virtually a full-time job, and now he is supported in his work there by the American Jewish Joint Distribution Committee (JDC), which was founded in 1914 as a relief agency to help Jews in trouble all over the world but from its inception rendered help to those in need regardless of religious affiliation.

Rick was still at Mother Teresa's when I found him that day, seeing patients and doing his daily "walk-through," his way of appearing in each dormitory in case somebody wants to bring a problem to his attention. When I told him about the little boy I'd found and described his deformed back, Rick hesitated for no more than a nanosecond before he said, "Let's go find him"—as if he didn't already have enough work to do with the hundreds who wait in line to see him. He takes on new cases with gusto, so much so that even on the odd Sunday when he's out hiking and sees a fellow with a bad back, he actually stops the man and tells him to come to the clinic.

His patients—some are among those living at Mother Teresa's; others make their way from the barren countryside or the dusty villages that make up Addis Ababa—wait and wait for hours on end, without complaint, for a chance to have a consultation with the doctor, which in some cases will save their lives, in others, relieve them from constant pain. Some of the sickest kids who are housed at the mission roll themselves around in wheelchairs, while others stand about hoping for nothing more than a high five from the doctor. One teenager in a wheelchair crochets and sells colorful caps and carries an x-ray that he keeps showing to Rick, hoping for a new—and more favorable—diagnosis for the ailment that is crippling him.

As soon as Rick finished with his last patient, he and I and Berhanu, Rick's Ethiopian man Friday, who is himself something of a miracle worker, piled into Rick's beat-up Suzuki and drove to the place, in front of Florida Pastry, where I had seen the boy. It was a beautiful day, and the air in the eight-thousand-foot altitude of the city was sparklingly clear. Hundreds of pedestrians were still making their way down the street (the Ethiopians describe this as going "by leg"), but when we got to Arat Kilo, the boy was gone.

We asked some of the shoeshine boys nearby if they knew where we could find the child. They directed us to his neighborhood around the corner, but there was no sign of him there either. While my heart sank, Berhanu found a young man named Yeshetilla—which means "the great protector"—whose brother had been treated by Rick. Berhanu asked him to call if he saw the boy. We didn't have to explain whom we were talking about—everyone in the neighborhood seemed to know him.

We drove back to the clinic down broad avenues divided by medians full of sturdy weeds and passed flocks of goats being herded to the slaughter and donkeys with their burden of fresh-cut firewood. Addis is a fascinating city, but I was now too edgy to focus on the scenery; I was worried that we'd lost "my" boy—for that's how I'd started to think of him. As we were pulling up to the clinic, Berhanu's cell phone rang.

"That's him," I said, practically jumping up and down like an excited kid.

As Berhanu listened to the caller, a gentle smile spread across his face.

"How did you know?" he said.

Rick steered the Suzuki back to the appointed spot, and there he was, standing on a side street with Yeshetilla, ready to squeeze into the car. The boy did not hesitate for a moment, almost eager to set off with a bunch of strangers, and not just strangers, white foreigners. He was still wearing the same dirty green T-shirt, and now I noticed that the worn soles of his sneakers were flapping loosely from the tops. He struggled mightily to keep the dark jeans he wore from falling down.

He said his name was Danny—as with most Ethiopians, last names don't matter—and that he lived on the street. Yeshetilla told us—only somewhat correctly—that each night Danny paid the equivalent of ten cents for a place on the floor of a video store—nothing more than a flophouse—with about twenty older vagrants who smoked and chewed khat and where lice and fleas and rats feasted on all of them. He also said that Danny was about seven, maybe even eight, but not four. So the first diagnosis was easy: in addition to the hump on his back, he was suffering from malnutrition.

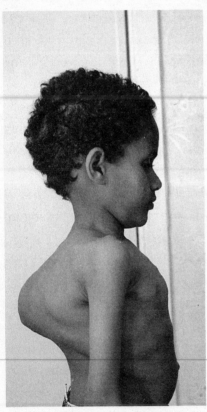

Danny, photographed by Rick, on the day he was found on the streets of Addis Ababa.

We returned to the clinic once again, where the first thing Rick did was to ask Danny to stand in front of a bare white wall so he could take his photograph, just as he does with all of his patients. In addition to a profile of his back—which was even more severely deformed than I realized when it was covered by his shirt—Rick wanted a picture of his face. He told the boy he had to smile.

"Doctors always ask why I send photos, why I don't just send the x-rays and blood studies," Rick said. "I want them to know this is a human being," he explained. "This isn't just a back. This is a soul."

Those photos are sent along with the lab work to Rick's contacts around the world; some will offer to perform surgery, some will confirm his diagnoses and provide advice on proper levels of medication. Others will send money.

Once Rick finished taking the pictures, he reached for his stethoscope, the only piece of medical equipment he has (if you don't count the Toyota key he uses to roll back eyelids and check for trachoma), and listened to Danny's lungs. He then tells the boy he's been having chest pains and puts the stethoscope in Danny's ears. Would the boy please check his heart?

"You're the doctor; I'll be the patient," Rick told him.

This got a big smile. It works every time.

Then, holding Danny by the shoulder with his free hand, Rick placed the stethoscope at various places on the boy's lungs, listened intently, and then looked up at me over his glasses.

"Marilyn," Rick said gently, "you've just saved a life."

If I was smitten before, now I was in love.

Had Danny gone untreated, which was practically guaranteed if he stayed on the street, his condition would have become critical. What he was suffering from, tuberculosis of the spine, would have caused him to become even more misshapen and crippled, like many of Rick's patients, and he would have been in ever-increasing pain. Within two years, Rick said, Danny's spine would collapse, damaging the spinal cord and causing paralysis. Lung function would slowly decrease and an excruciating death would follow.

Rick noticed that the boy was breathing very rapidly. "It's really important that we take care of him," he said. "If you're paralyzed in Ethiopia, and you can't move, you can't beg, and if you can't beg, you can't eat."

Rick got a kick out of my correct walk-by diagnosis of Danny's problem, which I was able to do from having observed him in the clinic. "Here one week and you've become a specialist in a disease few doctors in America have ever seen!"

This kind of tuberculosis—spinal spondylitis—is virtually unknown in the United States, and doctors who come to Ethiopia are at a loss to diagnose it.

DANNY IS ONE OF THE THOUSANDS in Ethiopia who suffer from diseases such as spinal TB or severe scoliosis. Some conditions are caused by birth defects; others, from severe malnutrition, infection, and lack of medical care. It is not rare to see these people on the street, their backs seriously distorted, some of them so crippled they can barely walk.

Ethiopia, once known as Abyssinia, is one of the world's oldest countries and a cradle of the human race, containing humanity's most ancient traces. It is rich in history and has more UNESCO world heritage sites than any other country. But in everything else, it is the poorest country in Africa but one, subject to periodic drought with all sorts of distribution problems. Medical care was hardly a priority under the famed Haile Selassie—certainly not for ordinary people—and it did not become a priority under the successive Communist government or the one after that.

Today the country has fewer than three physicians for every forty-five thousand inhabitants, but most of them are not in the public health service. Just one of many discouraging medical statistics illustrates how serious the doctor shortage is: 119 out of 1,000 babies die before they are five years old. Rick says there are more Ethiopian doctors in the Washington, D.C., area than in their entire homeland. That is why the diseases Rick sees have reached almost untreatable levels by the time patients get to him.

UPON COMPLETING DANNY'S PHYSICAL EXAM, Rick asked Yeshetilla, who was an old hand at navigating the medical system after caring for his brother, to take Danny for x-rays and blood tests the following day. Rick gave Yeshetilla money to buy dinner for the two of them and sent Danny back to the neighborhood where we found him. I was surprised that Rick didn't arrange for Danny to stay in a safe place right away, but he explained, "I don't feel it's right to grab a kid off the street precipitously, just like that."

The tests confirmed everything Rick had suspected. The x-ray—which Rick read by holding it up to the sunlight—showed tuberculosis of the lung and the spine, and the blood tests revealed malnutrition (this seven-year-old weighed no more than thirty pounds), iron deficiency anemia, and worms, which are very common. They are so common, in fact, that when Ethiopians are sick, they say "my worms are not eating." They think worms are a normal part of the anatomy that transform food and drink into waste and may become angry if the person doesn't eat properly.

Once Rick had the test results, he put out a call for Danny to come back to the clinic, but the message came back that Danny was too busy. He was watching a video, and it was not convenient for him to come. Among other things, Rick wanted to give Danny some hard-boiled eggs, and he'd put a few in his pocket that morning. Twenty minutes later he ran into an old friend who gave him an enthusiastic Ethiopian hug—a tight shoulder-to-shoulder three-kiss embrace. So much for the eggs. At least they were cooked.

Within days, Danny turned up, and Rick started him on the medicines he needed. He found a place for him to stay in a dormitory at Mother Teresa's, where the beds abut each other side to side and end to end with just enough space between them for the kids to sidle through. This bed, one of hundreds of cots neatly made up with matching flowered quilts, was the first real one Danny ever had. Now he was safe and sheltered from the elements and surrounded by other boys, some orphans, others with the usual array of problems from heart disease to cancer.

But Danny was not a happy boy. He told us that the next day was Timket, the holiday that commemorates the baptism of Jesus, and like many Ethiopian holidays, a day particularly profitable for beggars. Yet here he was, stuck inside, missing out on a big payday.

"I talked to him at length," Rick said, "about how I want him to have a bright future and to help him go to good schools. He was a bit okay with that, but still bummed to be away from his street-boy friends. The people in his village are delighted that he's off the street and has more of a future."

It didn't take long for the little boy to adjust to the good life. "Danny, did you have a shower?" Rick asked him a few days later. "Yes, with warm water," Danny replied, his eyes wide with amazement at this new luxury. He also found out what it is to wear clean clothes and shoes that are not falling apart, to eat three meals a day, and to have the companionship of the other boys.

In the days ahead, he especially seemed to thrive on his daily outings with Rick, who became as taken with him as I was. They'd walk hand in hand to the juice store down the block, where Rick drank his usual—a rainbow parfait of avocado, banana, guava, and papaya layered with a dash of grenadine, his entire lunch. It was on these outings that Danny discovered the pleasure of warm milk and cake at the adjacent Italian coffee bar, one of the many reminders of the brief Italian attempt to colonize Ethiopia. The Italians didn't last long—only five years—but they left a tasty legacy of macchiato, pizza, and spaghetti. And the word *ciao* has been incorporated into the Ethiopian language.

One day as Rick and Danny were making their way down the street, the boy stopped for a moment and looked up at Rick. "Let's hop," he suggested. So there they were, Rick, in his striped button-down shirt and khakis and baseball cap and Danny in his mission-issued (clean) hand-me-downs, hopping along on the rubble of stones that passes for a sidewalk, holding hands and laughing their way to the kiosk. It was just about the first kid thing the boy had ever done.

Earlier that week, Rick had said to no one in particular, "I've got half a mattress free." This meant that there was a small bit of unused space at the house he shares with the horde of children who have become his family. Some of these kids are patients who have already undergone surgery, like Dejene and Zewdie, whose crippled backs were repaired, and Mohammed, who lost a leg to cancer and now wants to become a cancer researcher. Others, like Tesfaye and Zemenewerk, are still awaiting their operations. Some made their way alone from the countryside and had the good luck to find Rick; others were abandoned by their families and left on the streets of Addis to fend for themselves until Rick found them. Recently, some girls were added to the mix when Rick took in two spinal patients and then Zewdie's sister, Balemlai (whose name means "on top of the world"), because she was eager for an education, and then another when he literally bumped into Zemenewerk, a tiny twelve-year-old who was walking along the street in Gondar with her uncle, both of them in tears because the hospital had turned her away as a hopeless case.

These improbable encounters have led Rick to fill his conversations with references to God and miracles. He's convinced that some mysterious power keeps putting people in his way who need help.

"If you are not religious," he said recently, "you ascribe it to coincidence; if you are a believer, you attribute it to God."

Rick, who was born Jewish but of the three-day-a-year variety, became a modern Orthodox Jew when he was thirty-seven years old. Now he is completely convinced that God makes everything happen. Even my decision to walk that day instead of taking a taxi went into his miracle category because that's how I found Danny.

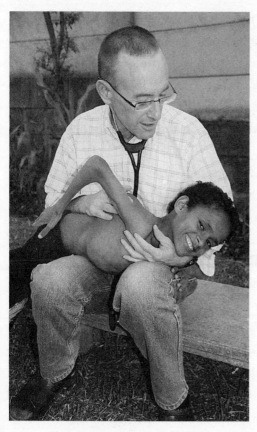

Rick checking on Danny's progress.

Rick is an enigma, although here the word seriously understates the case. From his early years, he seemed to be looking for a spiritual home, but that search was independent of and parallel to a compelling instinct to help those in need. He wasn't performing good works because the commandment enjoins us to do unto others. His altruism, it seems, was innate. For him it was normal to do good, and only later did he find in the Talmud reinforcement of his humanitarian instinct.

One day Rick invited Danny home for the weekend, but the boy hesitated. By then, he was happy enough at Mother Teresa's, and he'd already had enough change in his life. Still, one of the sisters encouraged him to go and he did, albeit reluctantly. Another weekend Danny was included in a Sunday family outing to Sodere, a scruffy resort where Mohammed, one of the older boys, carried him on his back in the swimming pool. Danny had even gotten strong enough to challenge some of the other kids to a race.

And then, a couple of weeks later, Danny went home to

Rick's for good. That "half a mattress" became his. It was like winning the Ethiopian sweepstakes.

Within two months of being rescued from the streets, Danny was enrolled at "Holy Angels," a Christian school that, like all schools in Ethiopia, does not teach religion. He loved his classes, and all shyness disappeared as he announced his daily achievements.

"Attention everybody," he would shout at the top of his lungs. "Attention . . . 1, 2, 3, 4, 5, 6," he would start counting and continue up to the hundreds, demonstrating his proficiency in arithmetic.

"He comes home and walks around the house counting to three hundred in English," Rick says admiringly.

Mostly he thrived on being the center of attention. Whenever Rick came home from work, Danny would jump in his arms and that's when the horseplay began, with lots of laughs all around. Rick started giving some thought to finding a family in America that might want to adopt Danny, and I asked how he could possibly give him up. Rick, in his typically cool and noncommittal manner, said only, "He's happy with us."

Danny was, indeed, instantly at home at Rick's, a perfect fit in a busy household filled with chaotic high jinks, fiercely competitive Monopoly, rowdy card games, serious homework, and stand-up dinners. Everybody crowds into the cramped kitchen where they fill their plates from large bowls of vegetarian grains and rice, vegetables, and pasta. At night, after a bit of CNN or the BBC or a soccer game (or MTV if Rick isn't around), the mattresses get rolled out, the stained couches fill up, and everyone retires for the night.

On any given day you can find these kids in the sunlit garden/

playing field/rumpus room outside the three-bedroom bungalow that Rick shares with all of them.

The day I arrived was particularly bright and beautiful— Ethiopia calls itself a land with thirteen months of sunshine— and the kids were all outside. Dejene (fully recovered from back surgery) was tossing a soccer ball to Mesfin (being treated for a growth-hormone deficiency) who smashed it to Mohammed (who lost a leg to cancer) who tapped it to Tesfaye (awaiting particularly complicated back surgery for TB of the spine). The passport into this group may be a life-threatening disease, but this is no rehab facility. In this one-story ranch-style house, Rick has made a home for these children and more than a dozen others. He treats them, feeds them, educates them, gives them shelter, and prepares them for a productive future.

These Ethiopians playing in the yard seem like fairly ordinary kids, but if it weren't for Rick, they might not be alive. They might be living on the street, like Danny was, or, if they were very lucky, inhabiting a dusty corner in one of the tin-roofed one-room shacks that are the main form of housing in the city or one of the conical thatch-roofed, windowless *tukuls* in the countryside.

Bewoket, now twenty-four, was near death when Rick saved him with hours of dedication and $10 worth of medicine. He was so gravely ill that Sister Tena at Mother Teresa's told anyone who would listen: "Dr. Rick is going to heaven no matter what he does in his life because no child was ever as sick as Bewoket was and survived here."

Rick took Bewoket in and discovered that it wasn't a terrible sacrifice to give up his solitary way of life. He started taking in other sick boys and eventually officially adopted five kids—the limit in Ethiopia—the first two because they needed surgery, which he couldn't afford. As part of his family, they were covered under his family health insurance plan. Until then, Rick was pretty much a loner, accustomed to living an uncharted life in which he had few obligations and could do whatever he wanted when he wanted. Except for a short stint on the wrestling team when he was in junior high school, he was never a team player; in high school and college he went in for individual sports like swimming and running—but never on a team. When he traveled, he traveled mostly alone. So he weighed very carefully what it would mean to make the life-changing commitment to bring children into his life.

"I had serious qualms," he said, "but I thought about it for five days before I realized that God was sending me a message: 'The Almighty is offering you a chance to help these boys. Don't say no.'"

Once he'd taken in Bewoket and then Dejene and Semegnew, the two boys who needed surgery, it was just a small step to bringing in the others—who now number twenty. The kids come from various parts of the country; they are Muslim and Orthodox Christian living in the home of an Orthodox Jew who encourages them to follow their own faiths and has no interest in converting them. He doesn't even want to make them into vegetarians, although no meat is served in his house as a way to keep it kosher.

One evening, in a rare moment when the house was quiet, Rick suddenly got it into his head to ask the boys a question:

"Hey, are we a family?"

Nobody had considered this. It's sort of like in *Fiddler on the Roof,* when Tevye asks his wife, "Do you love me?"

The kids looked around, then nodded. "Yeah, we're a family," they agreed.

"And are we happy?" Rick asked. "Yeah, we're happy," they said.

Dejene was the youngest at the time. "There's only two problems."

Uh-oh, Rick said to himself. "Dejene, what's the worst problem?" He looked up and said, "Farts."

"And number two?" Rick asked.

"Fights."

Rick pointed out that as a family unit, we're a lot happier than most families he knows in America.

It's hardly a "family" in the traditional sense, but these days there are more varieties of family than ever before. If the test of family is the care and affection one member feels for another, this one passes the test and might well be "happier than most."

2

A NORMAL DOCTOR?

THE HOUSE ON ANN DRIVE is just around the corner from Willits Elementary, where Rick and his two younger brothers went to school. When the family moved to this quiet, leafy, and shingled subdivision in Syosset, New York, Rick was just old enough to start kindergarten. The developer, it would seem, named the streets after the women in his family—Ann Way, Melanie Lane, Rita Street, Nana Place. Even a couple of boys, Donald and Stuart, were thrown in for posterity.

This new neighborhood was a small step up for the family from a tract house in the all-white community of Levittown, where Bill Levitt, a wartime Seabee, transformed acres of potato fields into America's first suburb with housing for returning World War II veterans. Built in an assembly line, the houses were spare but functional, and for $65 down, a vet could buy into the American dream, front lawn and all.

Rick was born on Memorial Day—that is, when it used to be celebrated on May 30—in 1953.

"I don't know what I weighed," he volunteers, "but you can't go wrong by saying 4.6 pounds."

He was a small but precocious kid with an unusually strong ability to memorize. In first grade he could recite the Gettysburg Address by heart, and his teachers started parading him around to all the classrooms to perform.

"Oh, no!" Rick moans. "Did my mother tell you that?"

She did, and Rick has a prodigious memory still.

"Don't tell Rick anything you don't want him to remind you of in twenty years," says a friend.

It's almost possible to discern a plan underlying Rick's journey from Syosset to Addis Ababa, but there was no road map.

The philosopher Martin Buber wrote that "all journeys have a secret destination of which the traveler is unaware." This was certainly true of Rick, who simply made his way from one adventure to the next, grasping at opportunities that had resonance to his soul. It can be satisfying now to overlay a template on his résumé and identify way stations that suggest a pattern where one event in his life led to another, but he was really more like an accidental traveler who serendipitously found his way to the surprisingly satisfying life he leads today.

By the time he was an adolescent, Rick was already becoming impatient with his life's everydayness. He was an excellent student and fairly bookish, and he tended to march to his own drummer. His younger brother, Dan, was the athlete in the family; Rick, the intellectual, although Dan said that Rick was a pretty scrappy member of the (bantamweight) wrestling team in junior high.

As a student at Syosset High, Rick was convinced that there had to be something more exciting than school, so every Saturday he started boarding the Long Island Rail Road; he traveled to New York City and found his way to the Henry Street Settlement House, where he was put in charge of tutoring underprivileged children. Not many teenagers looking for excitement would have chosen to tutor poor kids, but in Rick's case a philanthropic gene—or an altruistic heart—needed to express itself.

Rick also became known around his neighborhood as a pint-sized fund-raiser. Haunted by the images he was seeing on television, the bulging eyes and distended bellies of the starving children of Biafra, the breakaway province of Nigeria, Rick made himself a committee of one to raise money for the hungry. He was determined to draw people's attention to the civil conflict in that country that would leave more than a million people dead from war and famine.

"Rick definitely had a spiritual side," his brother, Dan, recalls. "While I was doing sports, he started to go to Quaker meetings. He was really curious and explored the faith quite carefully." His mother says he would get on his bike every Sunday and go to the Quaker meetinghouse, where the talk was of peace and justice and equality and the idea that we are all endowed with a measure of the divine spirit. And that wasn't all. He also went to midnight mass at Christmastime.

"He was looking everywhere," his mother said.

"He blossomed at an early age into cool stuff," Dan said.

We all think we're a long way from the circumstances of our youth, but Rick has stretched that distance farther than most. He was following a familiar path when he decided to go to Middlebury College, where he majored in geography, maybe because he dreamed of going to faraway places. As a child he was fascinated by the stories of Albert Schweitzer and Thomas Dooley, sometimes called the jungle doctor. He says it was a chance decision to major in geography but one that changed his life. In working on a study of the effect of climate on heart disease, he sought out Dr. Charles Houston, a professor of medicine and renowned mountain climber, and asked if he could work with him. Rick says they met in his office at the University of Vermont at least once a week for an entire year; Houston became his mentor. Days before Houston's death in 2009 at the age of ninety-six, Rick made a one-day trip to Vermont for a last visit to the man who became a major force in his life.

"Now," he says, "thirty-four years later, I still cherish that relationship. I may not have become a doctor if he had not encouraged me."

But as an undergraduate Rick still had no plan. For his junior year, he went to Fairbanks, Alaska, to study geography and Japanese—which was quite unusual in those days—and then hitchhiked south to California, where he joined a friend from Middlebury to trek the entire John Muir Trail, a 211-mile journey through high peaks, granite cliffs, canyons, and mountain lakes from Yosemite Valley to Mount Whitney. The journey became something of a head-clearing experience; as he wandered he weighed the possibilities for his future. He would determine his own path; never once did it occur to him to ask his parents for advice or permission.

His mother, Betts, with a good measure of understatement, says he did not consult with the family very often on anything. "From the day he was born," she says, "he was his own man. He's done everything on his own. He did what he wanted to do, and everything he did was right. Since nothing he did seemed wrong I had nothing to complain about. He never ceases to amaze me."

What makes a boy into a Rick? I looked to his mother for an answer. "I haven't the slightest idea," she says. Along the evolutionary timeline, it is theorized that humans became altruistic at about the same time man started to walk, some four million years ago. But it would appear that the DNA was not imprinted as deeply on every individual as it was on Rick.

Over the last couple of decades an entire academic industry has developed to examine altruism in the human species. Philosophers, biologists, and sociobiologists have been seeking to understand what evolutionary mechanism might explain the roots of altruism, and they have sought clues from studies of species as diverse as ant colonies, the honeybee hive, vervet monkeys, and chimpanzees. Darwinian natural selection comes in for some credit, as does a theory of group selection, in which case Rick's altruism would be explained by processes that occurred in the many generations of his family that preceded him. Of course Rick's lifestyle choice—at least so far—suggests that he will not be passing along his altruistic genes, much like the Medal of Honor winner who falls on a grenade.

Professor Edward O. Wilson, the world-renowned entomologist and curator of the Harvard Museum of Comparative Zoology, differentiates hard-core altruists like Rick, who expects nothing in return to himself or honor for his family, from the soft-core altruists, who are doing good because they expect honor or the satisfaction of other desires in return. It's a puzzlement, so much so that Stanford Medical School has started the Center for Compassion and Altruism Research and Education to "employ the highest standards of scientific inquiry to investigate compassion and altruism." The center states as its mission:

> To undertake a rigorous scientific study of the neural, mental and social bases of compassion and altruistic behavior that draws from a wide spectrum of disciplines including psychology, neuroscience, economics and contemplative traditions.

> To explore ways in which compassion and altruism can be cultivated within an individual as well as within the society on the basis of testable cognitive and affective training exercises.

A banner on the center's website says, "Imagine if we could tap into the part of the brain that makes us altruistic and compassionate." Perhaps Rick should allow them to scan his brain. I'm sure a PET scan would show that the pleasure area of his brain lights with activity when he is able to help someone. That's what makes him happy.

Rick is perplexed when asked why he does what he does, living in uncomfortable conditions, taking in kids with all manner of disease, forswearing his own progeny. Zvi Kresch, a medical student who was one of the volunteers who spent time with him, says, "He has a very deep-rooted moral compass. He looks at how he can affect certain circumstances regardless of whether or not it's the best thing for him. It's not within Rick's realm of understanding to turn your back on need."

Rick acts as if his kind of selflessness were an everyday commodity that requires no explanation.

"I don't think I'm doing anything special or that I'm an unusually good person," he says. "I just like to help people. Once you see what the need is, I just don't see how you cannot do this. I'm simply trying to do good work and be a decent person."

Rick lives his life by Albert Schweitzer's principle that "you must give some time to your fellow men. Even if it's a little thing, do something for others—something for which you get no pay but the privilege of doing it."

Rick graduated from Middlebury in 1975, still unsure about what he wanted to do with his life. He hitchhiked back to Alaska, where he found a job on the night shift in the supply room of a hospital. Quiet evenings gave him a chance to read and to have long talks with the doctors on duty. These surroundings, bolstered by his experiences with Dr. Houston, inevitably led Rick to thoughts of medical school, so—just in case—he signed up for a premed program in Alaska. But at this point he also began to veer sharply off the customary pathways of a child of suburbia. In those days, hardly anyone thought of taking a gap year to go off and explore the world. Although some form of teenage rebellion was as common then as it has been ever since the time of Socrates, it was not the norm to take a journey into the unknown.

Rick became a pioneer of sorts when he went off on his own on the first of three trips around the world, toting a sleeping bag and living on a few dollars a day. His grandmother called him a "vagrant." His early travels took him to Hawaii, Burma, Thailand, India, Bangladesh, and Kosovo as well as parts of Africa. Confronted with the misery and poverty and epidemics and famine in so many countries, he became convinced that as a physician he could best start to deal—one by one—with the ills of the world. That became even clearer when he visited Calcutta.

There he drank in India's ancient culture with its occasional pockets of considerable wealth surrounded by crowds and chaos, poverty and suffering, pollution, hunger, homelessness, and despair. Overwhelmed by all of this, he decided he wanted to see Mother Teresa and took himself from his Salvation Army hostel to Kalighat, where she ran a home for dying destitutes.

"I entered a bit nervously and looked around," he recalled. "It was a large crowded room, quite clean, with several rows of cots holding men looking thin, emaciated, and sick."

He wasn't there more than a few seconds when a nun turned to him and, without a hello, said: "Bed number three didn't eat. Go feed him." He found his way to the porridge and started feeding the dying man, spoonful by spoonful, urging him to eat so he would gain strength.

"I wished I could do more," he remembered, "but I knew nothing about medicine, and feeding a few people was my task of the day."

He was told where he might see Mother Teresa and found his way to her house the next day. "I have a photo somewhere of the event, fifty or seventy women, dressed in white, chanting," he said. "I was impressed with their calm, their apparent simplicity, their happiness. Mother was there, one of the group. She did not stand out, except by her age. She had a kind, wrinkled face, was dressed identically to the others in a white sari with a blue stripe. Afterward I said hello and shook her hand."

He returned to Alaska, his decision to become a doctor now reinforced, and started sending out applications to medical schools. To pay the bills, he taught adult education classes.

When he went to Salt Lake City, Utah, for one of his medical school interviews, he put his backpack in a locker at the airport and carried his sleeping bag while he looked for a place to bed down for the night. He walked down the road from the airport until he found a field he considered acceptable— and a lot cheaper than a hotel—for a night's rest. Rick is very thrifty.

The next day he returned to the airport, retrieved his backpack, put on his suit to make himself presentable (if a bit wrinkled), and went to the interview. The admissions officer asked where he'd spent the night, and Rick said he'd slept in a field near the airport.

"But it snowed last night," said the school official.

"That didn't bother me," he replied. "I've been living in Alaska."

He was accepted at a number of medical schools, but chose the University of Rochester in New York because it offered what he considered a more humane form of medicine with greater emphasis on the doctor-patient relationship than on the diagnostic equipment that has mechanized the practice of medicine and created a gulf between physician and patient.

In a letter Rick wrote some years later to the *Texas Monthly*, he said it had taken him time to realize that his experience in Rochester was unique and that the training he had there had made him into the doctor he is today.

A primary goal of that training, he says, was to make an early connection to the patient. "All our rounds were at the bedside," he recalled, "and physical exam was greatly stressed. We watched with awe as faculty taught us to percuss (the motion is from the wrist, not the elbow), to listen, and ask the patient to say *eee*, to hear lung sounds, heart murmurs, to tap out the dimensions of the liver."

Rick remembers: "We once walked out of a patient's room and the attending physician asked, 'What kind of dog does this man have?' There had been no discussion of pets. We were dumbfounded. He sent a student in to ask if he had a collie. Sure enough, he did. 'How did you know?' we asked eagerly. 'Well,' he replied, 'he had a get-well card with a collie on it.' To paraphrase Osler, 'you can observe a lot just by looking.'"

Rick worries that American doctors no longer get that kind of training in interviewing or physical examination. When he went on to Johns Hopkins for his internship, he says, cases were discussed in a conference room, devoid of the patients.

"The rounds were intellectual, two-dimensional exercises, interesting but somewhat unreal," he remembers. "As we discussed causes of elevated bilirubin, we were disconnected from the human being who was ill, who had forgotten her reading glasses, who worried about her hospital bill and missing her daughter's wedding. She had inadvertently turned into 'the gallbladder in room 216.'"

Rick came face-to-face with the state of American medicine personally when he recently had to go for an examination following some abnormal blood tests, which fortunately turned out to be local lab error.

"In working these up on my last trip to the States," he recalled, "I went to a competent internist. . . . He sat with his back toward me, taking my history and typing into his computer. I felt like I was applying for a home mortgage loan, not beginning a session of healing."

The experience caused Rick to reflect on the fundamental importance of the physical examination and the way it helps the doctor and the patient to connect. He understands that in America there are considerations of insurance and time and money, but in Ethiopia, he likes to say, he has no financial concerns at all, except that he's giving away any money he has. But he knows his patients have been too long neglected, that they are afraid they will die, so he tries to find ways to comfort them, to show a little compassion, to buoy them up. He looks them in the eye and always tries to give them something to smile about.

"At the mission where I spend hours every day, I have nothing to rely on except my hands and a stethoscope," he says. "I wear it around my neck, only because I haven't owned a white coat in nearly two decades, and it doesn't fit into my pocket."

He says that whenever he teaches medical students in Ethiopia, where technology is far scarcer (there are a handful of CAT scans in this nation of more than 80 million), they are forced to rely on physical exam to come up with the diagnosis and this could make them far better doctors than their Western counterparts who run back to the machines.

"Ultimately," he wrote in the letter to *Texas Monthly,*

> *whether we are physicians in Austin or Addis Ababa, we're here to heal. When doctor and patient connect, the therapeutic relationship starts on a better foot with talking, listening, empathy, and with appropriate touching. The touching is vital. Speaking to the back of a typist filling in a form,*

*followed by a cursory listen to the heart and lungs
and a couple of quick depressions of the belly may
be faster, but it leaves the patient feeling unfulfilled
and slighted.*

There is a growing recognition in the medical community of the need to pull back from technology-driven medicine and instead to place greater emphasis on human interaction, although standard medical insurance that pays premiums for diagnostic procedures and not for time spent with a patient has inhibited the process. Doctors Eric J. Cassell and Mark Siegler, in their book *Changing Value in Medicine,* acknowledge that attempts to reorient the direction of the medical curriculum have not been very successful: "There are even some who feel that the problem has actually worsened." They note:

These commentators point out that in recent decades, medicine seems to have become increasingly technological and scientistic, and consequently more impersonal. According to that view, we take into our medical schools the most compassionate, concerned, and bright young people and turn them into "autotechnicons." While that may be a somewhat harsh viewpoint, it is certainly true that it is difficult to compete in the students' list of priorities with biochemistry or learning to do technical procedures or to read CAT scans.

Rick frequently quotes William Osler, the man who transformed American medicine. Osler was recruited to help estab-

lish Johns Hopkins Medical School at the end of the n
century, having literally written the book that was the underpin-
ning for medical education in the United States. He studied all
over the world and then adapted the best practices for American medicine, codified in his book, *The Principles and Practice of
Medicine,* first published in 1892. Rick was dedicated to Osler's
precept that "medicine is learned by the bedside and not in the
classroom. Let not your conceptions of disease come from words
heard in the lecture room or read from the book. See, and then
reason and compare and control. But see first . . . . If you listen
long enough, the patient will give you the diagnosis."

An internship in internal medicine and primary care provided
Rick with direct and intense contact with patients. He worked in
the Baltimore City Hospital, part of the Johns Hopkins network,
and in no time at all, he created trouble for himself when he had
the temerity to admit an eighteen-year-old African boy who had
congestive heart failure. What followed was a quick dressing-
down from the vice president, William J. Ward (now an execu-
tive in health-care and financial management), who demanded
to know: "Why was this patient not screened for insurance?"

Rick shot back an angry reply. "It is my understanding," he
wrote in a formal letter,

> *that we are to provide compassionate and
> efficient care to all, regardless of race, sex, religion,
> nationality, or insurance status. On numerous
> occasions in the emergency room, I have seen a
> physician tell a patient that he must be admitted
> and then the patient refuse, saying he has no*

*insurance. At that point the ER attending reassures
the patient and says, "Don't worry about money,
you need to be here for your own life and safety."*

*Sir, yesterday you pointed out to me "We are
not running a charity ward here," and said there
would be a lot of talking before this will happen
again. Is it now the policy of our hospital to only
admit sick patients who are fully insured? Would
you take responsibility for sending this patient out
of the ER?*

*You stated yesterday that you are always
"somewhat skeptical" of Sunday admissions because
"it is easy to sneak somebody in . . . Mr. Ward, I
sincerely felt this patient was acutely ill. . . . The ER
attending concurred. His condition was listed as grave.*

There is some irony in the fact that this occurred in William
Osler's own hospital, but the Hopkins medical staff was quick to
respond in accordance with Osler's principles. The chief of medicine, Dr. Philip Zieve, was so incensed that an administrator had
questioned the judgment of a doctor on his staff that he stepped
in immediately to back up Rick, saying, "If tomorrow one hundred uninsured Afghan refugees show up, I will admit each and
every goddam one of them."

Rick's willingness to stand up for those excluded from care
by the medical system was cited when he was nominated for a
prestigious medical award from the American College of Physicians.

Throughout his years in medical school, Rick continued to
travel whenever he could. The summer after his first year in

medical school he returned to Bangladesh, and in the middle of his fourth year he worked as a volunteer at the Christian Medical College in Vellore in the south of India. (Now the college has returned the favor by providing surgery for some of Rick's patients.) Whenever he was able to, he visited Mother Teresa's clinic in Kalighat, and on one trip contracted TB and had to take medication for a year to prevent the disease from becoming active.

"I would visit Mother Teresa's home, feed someone or wash a couple of people," he remembers. It was this attachment to Mother Teresa's work that would draw him to her mission in Addis Ababa.

Rick's father visited him when he was back in Baltimore, and one evening asked if he'd ever seen a patient die. "Dad," Rick replied, "when you work in the emergency room, you may lose five or six a day." But like all doctors, he coped, sometimes with grief, sometimes with black humor.

"As a senior resident teaching interns," he says, "I'd always explain that when someone dies, you speak with the family and ask two things: permission for autopsy and permission to donate eyes. The question always comes up 'What do you ask for first?'

"You can argue that either way, based on the value to humanity (eyes), the value to your own knowledge and other docs (autopsy), by what you think the family is most likely to agree to, etc. But I'd explain that in Baltimore, you always ask for eyes first.

"'Why?' they'd ask with curiosity.

"'Because if you get the eyes donated, you get free tickets to the Baltimore Orioles.'

"They would look at me incredulously, but that was the

end of the discussion. In fact, in the ER we'd often get someone with a heart attack, do CPR unsuccessfully, and then there would be a discussion among the interns. It would often end with 'Well, I already have eyes this month, so you can go inform the family.'"

Of course, Rick's attitude toward death is in no way as cavalier as this sounds. He has developed a form of armor that doctors use to shield themselves, he explains, because "you can't feel the pain too much. The biggest crisis in a decade for the family in front of you is one patient of eight on your checklist, and if you spend too much time with that patient or with that family, you'll never get out of the hospital."

Rick expressed his profound feelings about death and dying in a letter to a young medical student whose grandfather had just died.

"Every so often, I feel like I've done something right," he wrote.

At the end of a month on the solid tumor service of the Hopkins Oncology Center (which is divided, in medical slang, into solids and liquids, the latter being leukemias), one of my patients was a girl in her late 20's. She'd had non-Hodgkin's lymphoma for years. Great family, dad was an ex-military officer who had a crew cut who loved his family and loved his country.

Sharon was getting worse by the day, no longer responding to her chemo. We had nothing else to offer. She was exhausted and was sick, a bit out of it, tired of fighting all these years—tired of receiving chemotherapy, losing her hair, and tired of puking her guts out with chemo, tired of getting poked with IV sticks into her veins which were solidifying, and tired of being tired. In short, she was looking forward to the world to come, whatever that is. The family made her a DNR, do not resuscitate. An appropriate decision.

Good families do that. In my mind there is a time to realize that enough is enough. Fucked-up families say "I want everything done," a magical thinking move which in their minds might return their grandmother to them, just in case they decided to start speaking to her after all these years.

I had gotten to know that family pretty well, and I was going home after a night on call. I realized it was quite likely she would not be around in the morning—she was pretty much unresponsive.

As I was heading out of the hospital for the day, I called the parents out of her room for a moment. "Listen," I said, "I realize Sharon is really sick, and she's not long for this world. I just want to say good-bye to you folks, just in case." The father looked at me with tears in his eyes and said, "Thanks, doctor, for everything you have done." Actually, I was the baby on the team. Above me was an oncology fellow and an attending; they were the ones with the brains. I made no decisions, I just plugged in the IVs and did the blood tests and

*fever workups when she spiked fevers after chemo.
And I was the one who did spinal taps to instill
chemo into her spinal canal. But I was the one the
family got to know best.*

*I knew these were churchgoing folks. They had
no idea what religion I am. I said to them, "Would
you mind if I said a prayer with you folks?"*

"Doc," the father said, "that would be great."

*I'm sure her family had been praying for
healing for years, and there was no apparent
healing. So I simply said, "May G-d care for her
and her soul." Her father turned his eyes to me and
looked at me with a slight hesitation; I could tell he
was thinking about what I had said. He paused for
half a second, then nodded affirmatively.*

*I shook hands with everyone, including the
patient who was in a semi-coma, and slowly
walked out. At the door I turned and waved to
them and half winked, as if to say, "It's going to
be OK, whatever happens." She died that night, it
was the last time I saw them. That is the best of
circumstances.*

"Should we pray with our patients?" Rick asks. "As a med
student, politically correct leftist atheist (Jewish) residents used
to make fun of one of our Catholic attendings who would sometimes pray with the patients."

Rick was not one of them. He says he would ask himself, "How
would the patient feel about us praying? Or the family?" He said,

"In my experience, whites have mixed feelings. Blacks, they love to pray. Take a look at Horace Williams and his family:

"Horace, a decrepit Baltimore guy who had a stroke, could not walk, had very high blood pressure, and was largely bed-ridden. Horace would come into clinic once a month by ambulance, and I would take his blood pressure, talk with his wife and mother about his feeding and bowel movements, and adjust his meds.

"After a year or so, I knew them fairly well. And one day I said to them, "Can we pray?" Their eyes lit up. And we all joined hands and I'd say, "Oh Lord, please help Horace, he's not doing well, he lost his appetite, his blood pressure is up," and his wife would interrupt and say "and he's vomikin,'" and his mother would say, "he didn't eat nothing all day." And we'd go around and give everyone in the room a chance to say something to the almighty about old Horace, and I'd say, "And lord, please help him." I'd nod my head and we'd drop our hands, and look at each other and realize that somehow, we all felt a bit better. Who knows if it helped Horace, but it helped us.

"If one visits the sick but fails to pray for mercy he does not fulfill his religious duty."

During a five-week break from his internship in 1984, Rick volunteered to go to Ethiopia to assist during a devastating famine, the famine that prompted the worldwide Live Aid rock music concerts to raise money for the hundreds of thousands of people dying of hunger. At times, Rick was the only physician for ten thousand displaced people in a region devastated by a cholera epidemic. An estimated one million people eventually died of starvation.

Haile Selassie, the diminutive emperor of Ethiopia, along with his courtiers, had simply ignored the famine in the 1970s and did nothing to build up reserves of grain for future shortages like the one in the mid-1980s. Each successive period of famine left the population increasingly vulnerable to disease and the country less able to do anything about it.

In times of famine, the most effective way to prevent starvation and disease is to deliver food to the people where they live. But in this case the food arrived too late, and thousands had abandoned the countryside, leaving their crops and their dying animals behind, thereby exacerbating the shortfall. The people had left their lands and were starving to death.

Rick worked in a camp for mothers and children established in Wollo Province by Abie Nathan, whom he described as "the cantankerous, maniacal, impossible, but also truly caring Israeli peace activist." Although there were no Jews in the area where Rick was operating, his mission was underwritten by the Religious Action Center of Reform Judaism, based in Washington. Mother Teresa visited—the last time Rick got to see her—and asked Rick and his team to do what they could to ensure that the aid continue. Rick was struck that Mother Teresa's influence lay in the fact that while she chose to live with the poorest of the poor and not seek power, paradoxically she acquired great authority and became an important world figure. Rick had heard that the American ambassador in Addis Ababa was lobbying for more aid for Ethiopia and was having difficulty getting it approved. When Mother Teresa came to the embassy, he arranged for her to call the president of the United States to ask for more assistance.

"It worked," Rick said. "Ronald Reagan could not say no to Mother Teresa."

When Rick returned once again to Baltimore and completed his internship, he applied for a Fulbright grant to go anywhere in Africa—anywhere but Ethiopia, because he'd already been there. The Fulbright organization, however, had not sent anyone to Ethiopia since the Communist takeover in 1974 and wanted to reestablish a presence there. Rick's work during the famine made him a more valuable asset to the program in Ethiopia, so he was asked to go back. He returned for two and a half years to teach medical students and see patients at the medical schools in Gondar and Addis Ababa. He had no idea that this was to be the beginning of a much longer commitment.

The BBC World Service and his shortwave radio became Rick's link to the outside world in this pre-Internet era. On Saturday mornings, he tuned in to a sermon offered each week by Britain's most esteemed rabbi, Hugh Gryn, a Holocaust survivor. On each program the rabbi delivered the Torah portion of the week and offered a five-minute talk on the ethical underpinnings of Judaism that had universal application and appeal.

For Rick, the rabbi's messages were a revelation. A child of the Reform movement of Judaism, he and his family had observed the major holidays but not much more. He was still in search of a spiritual mooring. As a teenager he was already looking for answers at those Quaker meetings, which he attended with great seriousness and great regularity. But now, in Ethiopia, as he listened to the rabbi's words each week, he started to feel he might have missed something those many years ago when he studied for his bar mitzvah in a Reform temple in Long Island. Rabbi Gryn's broad intellectual and moral approach touched a chord in Rick and inspired him to delve into the deeper meaning of Judaism. When he returned to the States, he studied with a rabbi in Rockville, Maryland, and then at a yeshiva in Jerusalem.

As this process unfolded, Rick became an Orthodox Jew; his lifelong spiritual quest that began when he was a teenager was over.

He was attending Yeshiva Aish HaTorah in Jerusalem during the summer of 1990, when he began to hear about the plight of Ethiopian Jews. He decided he wanted to help—Rick never allows trouble to find him; he always goes looking for it. He posted a letter to the Jewish Agency in which he explained that he was a medical doctor, that he spoke Amharic, and that he had spent time in Ethiopia. Was there something he could do?

These credentials seemed almost too good to be true—that a Jewish doctor with experience in Ethiopia just materialized out of nowhere at the very moment when there was a growing medical emergency among Jews in Ethiopia. The Jewish Agency, which is normally in charge of immigration, forwarded his letter to the American Jewish Joint Distribution Committee, which quickly took him up on his offer and gave him a six-week contract to start on November 15, the limited appointment designed to give the organization an escape hatch if it didn't work out. But it did. His contract was extended another six weeks and now, nineteen years later, he is still there and still working with the JDC.

He was charged with overseeing the health of thousands of Ethiopian Jews who had converged on Addis Ababa expecting to leave immediately for Israel but who were held there in substandard and dangerous conditions for many months by the Marxist Ethiopian government, which was bargaining for something in return, mainly armaments to defeat a growing insurgency dedicated to overthrowing the regime. Rick quickly became an integral part of their community of hurriedly created refugee villages with health centers, schools, vocational programs, and even small businesses, which saw them through until they would be allowed to emigrate.

When the moment to leave finally arrived, Rick was given a ticklish assignment that demanded both medical and diplomatic skills: to extract the sickest patients from hospitals around Addis so they could be airlifted, along with the other Ethiopian Jews, to Israel. This one-day evacuation of more than fourteen thousand people, known as Operation Solomon, became the largest and fastest exodus in recorded history.

Rick's travels had by now taken him from Syosset to Alaska to India, Bangladesh, Israel, and Ethiopia, from medical residency to a land of famine that now faced an insurgency, and throughout his adventures, his grandmother Rose kept sending him hectoring letters in what he remembers as her curly script handwriting.

"When," she kept asking, "when are you going to be a normal doctor?"

3

TO SAVE A SINGLE SOUL

RICK DID BECOME A "NORMAL DOCTOR" ONCE, and for the only time in his life, when he returned to the United States after his Fulbright years. He joined a private group medical practice in Shady Grove, Maryland, which left him with enough time for study with a rabbi.

"I had a great job," he remembers, "low pay but great flexibility. I could set my own hours and take a week off with little notice."

He left the practice after a year and a half when he went to Jerusalem to continue his religious study at the yeshiva, and very soon after that, he was drawn back to Ethiopia when the JDC took him up on that offer to help the Ethiopian Diaspora.

The Ethiopian Jews, sometimes referred to as the "black Jews," are descendants of an ancient community whose origins are still obscure. They call themselves Beta Israel (House of Israel), but their neighbors called them *Falashas,* a derogatory term meaning exiles or strangers. The Amharic word can also be translated as "the landless ones." For centuries, Ethiopian law enjoined them from owning land, which made them a people set apart in a largely agricultural country. To support themselves they became artisans, creating exquisite pottery and jewelry.

There is no definitive history of how the Jews first came to Ethiopia. Some accounts suggest that the Ethiopian Jews of today may be descendants of the Hebrews who began their wanderings during the Exodus after they were expelled from Egypt and made their way to Abyssinia from southern Arabia. One legend suggests a royal lineage starting with the Queen of Sheba herself and her liaison with the great King Solomon. Ethiopian Christians believe that their son, Menelik, carried away the Ark of the Covenant, one of the holiest objects mentioned in the Bible, when he was in Jerusalem and brought it to Aksum, where it was revered ever after by the Christian community.

The Bible (Exodus) says that God commanded Moses to build the Ark to hold the tablets inscribed with the Ten Commandments. As the Jews wandered through the desert, the Ark was seen to have mystical powers to affect war and peace, plague and fire. Today, Ethiopian Christians hold to the belief that the Ark of the Covenant still remains in Aksum in the Church of Saint Mary of Zion, where a single monk, known as the Keeper of the Ark, guards the relic. There is, however, a competing legend, which places the Ark under the Temple Mount in Jerusalem.

Ethiopian Jews share some but not all rituals with their Western brethren. Their practices are taken directly from the Torah without reference to later commentaries of the Talmud, which shape the practices of Western European and Israeli Jews. They observe the Sabbath as well as Passover, Rosh Hashanah, and Yom Kippur; eat only meat from animals killed in accordance with Jewish law; pray morning and evening; and circumcise their male children eight days after birth.

As early as 1921, the JDC was looking into the welfare of the Ethiopian Jews, who had long been victims of anti-Semitism. Following a three-year study, the JDC petitioned Ethiopia's crown prince to assure their well-being. This was the first step into Africa for the JDC, whose guiding philosophy of social justice is based on the Jewish concept of *tikkun olam,* the moral duty to repair or heal the world. Equally strong is the tenet, attributed to Maimonides, that when you save a single soul, you save the world. Following these precepts, the JDC determined that when help was needed and it had the ability and the expertise, it would offer assistance, even if the contribution could be only a small part of the rescue effort.

The JDC started a program in Ethiopia in 1982 to provide support for Jews wishing to emigrate to Israel, but the schools, clinics, and water and agricultural projects it established, like its support for medical treatment at Mother Teresa's, were extended to non-Jews as part of its nonsectarian work.

When Rick, newly hired by the JDC, arrived in Addis on November 15, 1990, he found some twenty thousand Jews in desperate straits. They were dehydrated, malnourished, and suffering from pneumonia, tuberculosis, and various other diseases. Many of them had walked two hundred miles from Gondar and longer distances from other parts of the country because they were told they would be allowed to leave immediately for Israel. Instead, they were camped out for months in miserable conditions, a humanitarian crisis that, according to some, was created artificially by crowding these would-be emigrants into encampments that were so unsafe and so unhealthy that pressure would build on the government to expedite their departure.

To deal with the precarious conditions that resulted, the JDC set up an interim support program with schools and cottage industries and clinics operating seven days a week, twelve hours a day, with an impressive immunization program to minister to the refugees while the diplomats negotiated with the Ethiopian government for their release. The JDC support program brought down the death rate of the Ethiopian Jews from thirty-nine the first month to an average of three a month, below that of even Israel or the United States.

Rick, in effect, set up a public health service, which he said was successful because it emphasized health education, HIV prevention, nutritional support (deworming and vitamin A and iodine supplements), tuberculosis control, and general clinical care. The program also bolstered maternal and child health by providing financial incentives for mothers to deliver in hospitals. In addition, a program was instituted to train traditional birth attendants from inside the community to assist those who refused to go to maternity clinics.

The condition of the Jewish community was only slightly worse than that of the overall Ethiopian population, which was suffering severe hardship under the Communist government of Mengistu Haile Mariam. But now the Derg, as that government was called, was in retreat before the onslaught of the Ethiopian

Peoples' Democratic Alliance, a rebel group that was gaining ground in its battle to overthrow Mengistu. As province after province fell, Mengistu was looking for weapons anywhere he could find them, having lost his main sponsor with the collapse of the Soviet Union.

He turned to Israel as one source of military supplies and bargained for equipment with the Israeli envoys who had come to negotiate the release of the Jews. It soon became clear that Mengistu was playing on the fear that the Jews would be in danger as hostilities approached Addis and was holding the Jews hostage, allowing only about a thousand a month to leave. As Rick observed, "Letting all the Jews depart at once would be like killing the goose that laid the golden egg."

By May 1991, the rebel army was in walking distance of the capital, and Rick worried that if street fighting erupted, the Jews would become an easy target. Rick said at the time, "Nobody knew what would happen if the rebels entered the city; fierce fighting, cross-fires, bombing and napalm were all possible." He described the mounting tension: "There had been an explosion in the center of town. The rebels were rapidly approaching, and we all wondered how long this situation could continue. On Wednesday, the ubiquitous pictures of Mengistu started coming down, culminating on Thursday with the removal of the massive bronze statue of Lenin."

Mengistu finally faced the fact that it was all over for him and fled to Zimbabwe, where he has lived in exile ever since. (In 2008, the Ethiopian Supreme Court found him guilty of genocide and sentenced him to death in absentia.) Mengistu's departure was welcomed, but he left behind a dying country with one of the world's lowest per capita incomes and a population

increasing rapidly while food production was declining precipitously because of successive waves of drought.

Famine was a constant threat. Life expectancy was forty-one
years. More than 10 percent of Ethiopia's babies died within the
first year, and an additional 11 percent died before they were five
years old.

The Israeli envoy, Uri Lubrani, moved quickly to offer the
new government $35 million as an "incentive" to allow the Jews
to leave. Within two days, the deal was sealed, and word went
out to all the Jews seeking to emigrate: drop everything, bring
everyone in your families, as well as your embassy identification
cards and any medical records, and go immediately to the Israeli
embassy. The first planes were scheduled to depart for Israel in
the next twenty-four hours.

Rick was told to take an Ethiopian assistant and, without
attracting attention or allowing the operation to become widely
known, remove seven or eight patients from four different hospitals and bring them to the departure point. His role is but a foot-
note in the larger exodus, but his efforts that day to rescue sick
patients from their hospital beds and prepare them to embark is
emblematic of what he does still, every day—bringing hope, one
person at a time.

"I tossed all night," he remembered, "aware of the task we
faced."

He headed first for the leprosy hospital on the other side
of the city, to find Mandefro Alemo, a thin and frightened
thirteen-year-old suffering from both leprosy and tuberculosis.
Rick had seen him before and remembered that he was in the
bed at the end of the room. He pulled the blanket from over his

head and, using his limited Amharic, whispered to him to get up, that today he would go to Israel. The boy just lay there and cried.

"I walked out to the chart room to record his medications," Rick remembers. "While I was perusing his chart, his physician, a European, entered. I had known him casually several years before. I explained that the patient was under my care, and that we had a special flight for patients to Israel today and that he was eligible for this. This was as much information as I wanted to give out. Perhaps, I thought, it was too much.

"'No,' my colleague replied, 'he is under *my* care, and he is not going anywhere. And you have no right to see the chart. You are requested to leave here immediately, rounds are beginning.' I saw that there would be no compromise.

"One thing was for sure, Mandefro would not simply walk out of the hospital unhindered. I would not have minded kidnapping the patient, but this was virtually impossible with physicians, nurses, and hospital staff all nearby and my car parked 30 yards away. I considered coming back at night but had no idea how the rest of the day would go; I had many other patients to deal with, and the rebels could be in the city in the next 12 hours. I decided to go to the hospital director."

After a lengthy discussion, the director agreed to let the boy go, but since Mandefro was only thirteen, he needed permission from a parent or guardian. Rick suggested that the Israeli embassy was the ultimate guardian and asked if a letter from them would suffice. When he persuaded the director to accept a fax, Rick called the embassy where, unsurprisingly, he got a busy signal for fifteen minutes. Eventually somebody answered. Fine, he was told, but the fax is broken. "I again entered the director's office to explain the situation," Rick said, "wondering to myself what else could possibly go wrong."

Finally, the director agreed to speak to the embassy official. After what seemed like an interminable discourse about international standards of medical ethics, medical responsibility, and medical records, he finally agreed to give Rick a note to release the patient. Rick ran with it, literally. As he rushed about the hospital ducking orderlies and nurses he kept telling himself, "Remember, Ethiopians are good runners. You can't outrun an Ethiopian." He wanted to make his escape before any further roadblocks were put in his way.

"We entered Mandefro's ward," Rick recalled. "I simply told him 'Mandefro, *enehid ahun*'—let's go now. We lifted him out of bed and stood him up. He was too weak to walk on his own. I put his arm around my shoulder and we walked out. Halfway to the car, we were sighted by the staff. Wanting to avoid another long exchange, which would take more time and might challenge the decision of the director, I picked him up and ran with him to my car, leaving the director's note in the hands of a bewildered orderly. Mandefro was confused and crying, not comprehending what was going on. We put him in the back of the car, and as I pulled out, I ordered my translator to force him down on the floor and cover him with an overcoat.

"Fortunately, the guards had not been alerted, and we drove out without difficulty. As we entered the main road, I dodged military convoys, potholes, and animals as we explained to Mandefro that he would be leaving for Israel that day. He did not respond. About twenty minutes later, we arrived at our clinic.

I dropped the patient off and asked our nurses to take care of him."

It was already 11:00 A.M., and Rick had retrieved only one patient. He stopped at the Israeli embassy to grab some stationery with a seal, in case documentation was needed again, and headed for Yekatit 12 Hospital, where he was told a six-month-old boy had been in the emergency room for two days with meningitis.

Rick remembers: "I picked up the baby to do a brief exam. He had a low-grade fever, along with a slightly stiff neck, all consistent with his diagnosis of meningitis. I took the mother aside and told her quietly that there was an airplane that day that would take them to Israel, that we should leave immediately to prepare. She refused, speaking rapidly in Amharic that I found incomprehensible. I led her to a courtyard of the hospital and found an Ethiopian who spoke English. Perhaps, I thought, she doesn't understand my Amharic."

With the help of this new translator, he again tried to explain to the mother that a special flight was leaving that day for Israel, and she should get ready to go. Others overheard him, despite his effort to keep the operation secret, and said they too wanted to go to Israel. He had to explain to them why that would not be possible. They in turn urged the young mother to go, telling her the medical care in Israel is much better, but she continued to refuse, saying her brother had told her not to move and that he would meet her there at 1:00 P.M.

Rick explained: "Trying another approach, I informed the mother that at that very moment her brother was waiting for her at the Israeli embassy, and he had asked me to bring her there. It was an outright lie. In fact I had no idea who he was or how to contact him.

"I imagined that due to her stubbornness, she would be left behind. I was hot, thirsty, and tired, and frankly felt like strangling her. They teach you in medical school not to kill your patients, but I wanted to murder her.

"And I was uncomfortable with so many people knowing about this; even the knowledge of the special flight was not to be openly shared, but there had been no choice. The mother wavered for a bit, but then steadfastly refused to move. I considered simply disconnecting the IV and seizing the child myself, but this could be counterproductive. A crowd might start chasing me."

Totally frustrated by this time, Rick returned to the Israeli embassy. The streets were now teeming with Ethiopian Jews preparing for departure, a scene right out of the Bible where Jeremiah speaks of the people who will enter the Promised Land: the blind, the lame, women who were pregnant, women in labor.

"It reminded me of the Exodus from Egypt," Rick recalled, "fathers with sons on their shoulders holding one or two small children by the hand and perhaps a small suitcase or plastic bag with food. Their wives were next to them, each carrying a child on their back in traditional leather binders, holding another child by the hand, and carrying a bit of food."

Many of these people recognized Rick as he pushed his way through the crowd, stethoscope around his neck. Suddenly he was stopped by a man who was extremely agitated, crying, speaking quickly in Amharic.

"My sister and her baby are in the emergency room at Yekatit 12 Hospital. What should I do?" he asked.

Another miracle, Rick thought. "I smiled and told him, 'Let's go.'"

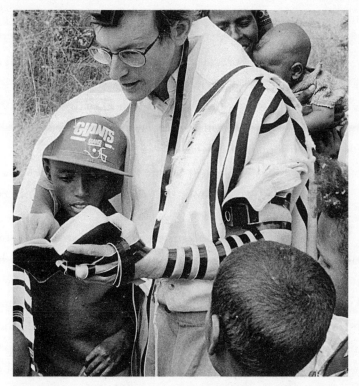

Rick at prayer with Ethiopian Jews as they prepare to leave for Israel.

When they returned to the hospital and the woman saw her brother, she agreed to leave immediately. Some of the nurses demanded that Rick check with the medical staff, but one of the doctors on duty turned out to be a former student of his, and they were on their way to the JDC clinic.

It was early afternoon when Rick returned to his office, which had now been transformed into a makeshift clinic, the floor covered with mattresses and IV fluid drips. He gave the child with meningitis an injection of a powerful antibiotic.

"We probably had the only supply in the country," Rick said.

Sister Tena reminded him that the people in the clinic were

hungry. "They have to eat," she told him. Rick had forgotten all about eating.

"This was May," he recalled. "In April we were sent ten thousand tons of matzoh, but because of clearances it arrived late, so it was still there. Sister got out the matzoh and to drink there was Slim-Fast that had been donated, nutritious but not exactly what the skinny Ethiopians required.

"I reflected that the Jewish people ate matzoh at the time of the Exodus from Egypt. Now they were again eating matzoh before this new exodus."

Earlier in the day, an exhausted and malnourished young man attempting to carry his wife, who was pregnant with her first child, had appeared at Rick's clinic. She was sixteen years old, had recently had malaria, and was severely anemic. Her husband told Rick they had traveled from Gondar to a Sudanese refugee camp in the hope of getting to Israel. He said they spent a year there before they left in frustration, walking the twenty-three hundred miles back to Gondar and then another two hundred miles to Addis.

Upon seeing this unfortunate couple, Rick became uncharacteristically annoyed. "My initial reaction was anger," he admitted. "I had hoped to take a nap, but looking at her, haggard and debilitated, I told myself to get to work and stop the self-indulgence."

He knew she would die without a transfusion, which meant she would have to be hospitalized, adding still another patient to the list of people he would then have to get to the airport and to Israel.

The husband weighed only a hundred pounds himself and was too weak to carry his wife, so Rick picked her up as best he could and carried her to the gynecology ward of Yekatit 12

Hospital, stopping every twenty or thirty yards to rest. To get a transfusion in Ethiopia one must first donate two units to the national blood bank, and for a donor to be accepted, he or she must weigh at least 110 pounds. Rick realized that there was no way the husband could be a donor, so the only option was to give his own blood. He frequently donated blood for his patients and was ready to do so again, but since he could give only one unit, an additional donor would also be needed.

"I stopped at the Hilton but was unable to find anyone I knew," he said. "A Canadian reporter who had previously promised to help begged off, saying he was waiting for a long-distance phone call. I asked a street boy who shined shoes to donate blood, promising him 30 birr ($15), a month's earnings. He agreed to at least come along and then decide." The street boy watched nervously as Rick's blood was taken and quickly changed his mind. Ethiopians look upon blood donation the way Americans think of parting with a kidney. Rick gently explained to him that a woman might die if he didn't help, but the boy said he didn't know her so it wasn't his problem. Rick returned to the Hilton lobby, desperate to find another donor. He saw an Israeli reporter he knew and appealed to him for help. The reporter said he couldn't, that he would be tired and weak for the next three days.

At that, Rick exploded, his voice filling the cavernous lobby. "Dammit, doesn't anyone give a shit? There is a pregnant woman dying, and you're worried about being tired tomorrow."

Rick ran out the door and the reporter—whose own wife was pregnant at the time—ran after him, shouting that he would be a donor. With a voucher for two units of blood, the pregnant

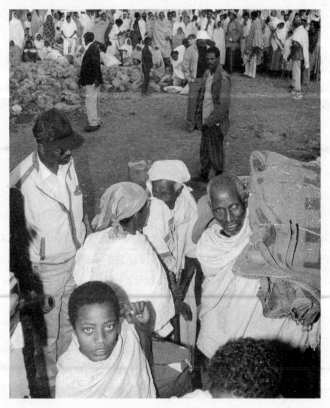

Ethiopian Jews massing to leave for Israel in Operation Solomon.

woman would get the transfusion she needed. Rick was relieved. "I thought she would survive the night," he said.

For the rest of the day and the next morning, Rick went from hospital to hospital, each with its own obstacle course of red tape, and eventually succeeded in collecting all the patients, including a woman with hepatitis who'd had a spontaneous abortion in the hospital, as well as a pair of twins who had been born prematurely.

The Israeli planes were about to arrive to begin the exodus. As he drove back to his clinic, Rick remembered, "I looked into the sky to see two long rows of solid white clouds with bright blue sky in between. Immediately, the parting of the Red Sea came to mind. Previously the Jews had departed through the sea; tomorrow it would be through the sky."

Throughout the night of May 24, 1991, forty-one planes from the Israeli Air Force and El Al, and one Ethiopian aircraft, all with their seats removed, landed and took off from Addis Ababa's Bole Airport carrying the Ethiopian Jews to Ben Gurion Airport in Tel Aviv.

One 747 boarded with 1,079 people, but landed with 1,080; a baby had been born prematurely just before takeoff. Of the remnants of hundreds of thousands of Jews centuries before, 14,310 were transported to Israel in the largest civilian airlift in history, going from war-torn Ethiopia to new lives, thrown into massive cultural changes overnight.

"Miraculously," Rick noted at the time, "despite the hordes of people, despite dehydration, malaria, appendicitis, women in labor and hospitalized patients, nobody had died. I was driven to the airport and got out on a supply flight filled with spare tires and aircraft parts. As soon as we took off, I fell asleep on one of the bunks on the wall and woke up as we were approaching southern Israel.

"As I stepped off the plane at Ben Gurion Airport, I recalled the period of the Gulf War in Ethiopia. The black Jews all had relatives in Israel and were quite worried about their safety. Every day we had started tuberculosis clinic with a roundup of the latest news gleaned from the BBC that morning. After the news, I would ask the patients to stand up and offer a prayer for Israel and for the soldiers in the Gulf. While many of us are self-conscious about praying in public, the Falashas would im-

mediately stand erect, lift their fingers in the air, and start spontaneous conversations with God. At one point, I turned to my
health assistant and asked him what the patient in front of me
was saying.

"'She is quoting from a psalm,' he replied. 'She is saying,
"The God of Israel never sleeps."'"

Here, once again, with their fingers pointed to the heavens,
these Ethiopian refugees on the tarmac were repeating their
prayer, now in their new homeland.

On his visits to Israel, Rick kept tabs on his patients. The
pregnant woman who almost died for want of a transfusion was
living on the top floor of a hotel in Netanya. Mandefro Alemu
was hospitalized in Jerusalem and was doing well. One month
after his arrival, he was reunited with his grandmother, his
guardian. The newborn twins were in good health and living
outside Haifa.

WITH THE EXODUS SUCCESSFULLY COMPLETED, Rick returned to
Ethiopia to oversee the JDC clinics for the remaining Jews in
Addis Ababa and Gondar. Every week or so Rick flew up to
Gondar, where the clinics were at the bottom of the highest hill
in the city and Rick's hotel, the Goha, was at the top. The walk
between the two provided him his daily exercise and a chance to
patronize the peddlers along the route by buying whatever they
were selling. He likes to encourage enterprise.

He always looked for Tilahun Molla, who, he knew, could
easily beg on the street but instead supported himself by selling

soap and plates and individual packets of tissue to passersby.

"He is a thin fellow, thirty or thirty-five years old, always smiling," Rick said. "He is a bit disheveled; his bodily hygiene could use improvement. He has marginal intelligence. He is frequently teased by local street boys, but is never perturbed. I believe that he is incapable of sin, and I consider him a sort of an angel."

Rick was a regular customer of another peddler as well, a woman who is blind, had been raped, and was left with a child. He always buys soap from her too, a lot of it.

At each of his regular stops, Rick would buy whatever was on offer: a bag of oranges, a kilo of bananas, soap, or "soft" (the generic name for any brand of paper tissues or napkins). Then, on his way back up the hill to his hotel, he would distribute his new purchases. Children, and occasionally even some grown-ups, would follow close behind to collect whatever he was handing out. The day he had the most fun was when he got hold of some kites and flew them as he ran up the hill, children skipping and scurrying after him. He looked like a benign Pied Piper.

One of the clinic patients in Gondar brought with her another of the amazing stories that seem to come only to Rick. She was in Quara, a pregnant woman dying of malaria. (Malaria in pregnancy is especially dangerous.) The nearest hospital was more than a hundred miles away, and there was no way to get there. Clearly she was going to die.

Then, as Rick tells it, for the first time in history, a military helicopter flying overhead had an engine problem and landed in her village. The villagers approached the crew, and they agreed to fly her to Gondar. "She was hospitalized, needed blood transfusions (I gave my blood to her), and delivered twins. They made it to Israel." Rick did not add that she named one of the children after him.

The Jews of Quara lived so deep in the countryside, so cut off from their brethren, they did not know of the exodus. Some years after Operation Solomon, the JDC sent special emissaries to their region to tell them they could now go to Israel. In time, they made their way to Addis, on foot. Some of the women gave birth along the way, got up, and kept walking. Among them was also a woman who they said could prove she was 110 years old. "God wanted her in Israel," Rick said. She lived there another six months.

When Rick examined the Quara Jews in Addis, he said he was the first white person these people had ever seen. "They weren't even sure I was a human being," he said. He spoke Amharic, so they thought well, maybe he was. "But his hair was not human," they told him. "They thought it was goat hair." Rick said that while he cared for them in the weeks before they left for Israel he spent time with them and taught them Jewish dances. They taught him Ethiopian dances.

"One day some of them came into my office," he said, "and saw the cover of a *Newsweek* magazine lying on the floor with a picture of members of the Ku Klux Klan holding hands in a circle. 'Look,' they said, 'Americans are dancing the hora and singing "Hava Nagila"!'"

Rick had now settled into a routine. He'd visit the clinics in Gondar and Addis and make occasional forays into the countryside to minister to the sick. He'd make trips to Israel and to the United States on fund-raising tours for the JDC. But even before he himself realized it, Rick was becoming only a visitor to the United States and a full-time resident of Ethiopia. He was a respected teacher of medical students, a distinguished doctor at the hospital, and about to become a father figure to a houseful of kids, most of them with serious medical problems, all of them lucky. It started with Bewoket.

4

AN ACT OF KINDNESS

By 1994, RICK HAD BEEN AROUND the Addis medical community so long that he pretty much knew everyone and they knew
him. As a Fulbright scholar, he had taught many of the doctors,
and his work at the JDC clinics and during Operation Solomon
had made him a familiar figure who was always welcome in the
wards. One day, while giving a visiting physician a tour of Black
Lion, the city's main teaching hospital, he came upon one of the
nurses he knew well and asked her whether there were any interesting cases to see.

"Oh yes," she replied. "You're a cardiologist, so you'll be interested in Bewoket. He tells us he walked to Addis Ababa from
Gojjam Province, about three hundred kilometers away."

The nurse led them to a room with nine beds, each one occupied by a child. For the benefit of the visitor, she described the three classes of care in this hospital: a first-class private room cost 30 birr (about $4.75 a day); a second-class two-bed room cost 11 birr ($1.75 a day), and a bed on a ward with eight to sixteen other people cost just over 2 birr, or about 35 cents U.S. The ward they were entering was for the poorest people.

"The Ethiopian tolerance for suffering constantly amazes me," Rick was telling his visitor as they made their way through the dingy hallways and past the emergency room. "Without frustration or complaint, Ethiopians sit with quiet dignity for hours in hot, stuffy, and dirty hospital rooms, only to receive far from optimum care."

On arriving at the children's ward to see the young cardiac patient, the nurse pointed to her right and said, "He is Bewoket." The doctors saw a boy about twelve years old in a tattered blue-and-white hospital gown, an Orthodox cross hanging from his neck. He was breathing rapidly, in obvious distress, sitting bolt upright with a torn piece of IV tubing taped to his nostril on one end and at the other to an oxygen tank.

The nurse removed an x-ray from the rusty metal bedside table and handed it to Rick. The boy's heart was more than twice the normal size, and he was clearly in severe heart failure, probably, Rick assumed, the result of rheumatic fever. Bewoket was suffering from a combination of ailments rarely seen any longer in the United States. At one time entire wards in America were filled with cases of rheumatic fever, a consequence of strep throat. These days, in the developed world, strep is cured in a day with antibiotics. In the third world, it is aggressive and often left untreated, causing complications that can lead to early death.

"When I arrived in Addis Ababa in the mid-1980s to teach at the medical facility," said Rick, "I was assigned the job of running the cardiac clinic, lecturing to the students about heart disease and consulting on cardiac cases on the wards. I was challenged with a new spectrum of disease with which I had little experience. I went back to the textbooks every night to read about what I saw on the wards, and within a couple of months I could successfully diagnose most patients using only my hands and my stethoscope.

"In Ethiopia, echo machines are very rare, and one practices middle-of-the-century medicine, relying only on the stethoscope and what lies in between its earpieces. A good doctor here will listen, percuss, and palpate. He will have the patient sit forward and listen to the heart at several points on the chest, and then have him lie on his left side and listen again. He will feel for the vibratory "thrill" of a heart murmur, the collapsing pulse and "pistol shots" over the arteries in aortic regurgitation, and the transmitted vibrations of aortic stenosis radiating into the carotid arteries of the neck."

Rick was always reminding his students that they could become better clinicians than their American counterparts because they are forced to use their eyes, ears, and hands to arrive at a diagnosis instead of being dependent on machines, which are rarely available in Ethiopia anyway.

As for Rick, he was learning how to deal with patients who came to him with an entirely new set of attitudes toward their own health, a process that made him a more sophisticated doctor. He chronicled the lessons learned some years later in an article for the *Western Journal of Medicine*, "Cross-cultural Medicine and Diverse Health Beliefs: Ethiopians Abroad," published in 1997:

To Ethiopians, health is an equilibrium between the body and the outside. Excess sun is believed to cause mitch ("sunstroke"), leading to skin disease. Blowing winds are thought to cause pain wherever they hit. Sexually transmitted disease is attributed to urinating under a full moon. People with buda, "evil eye," are said to be able to harm others by looking at them. Ethiopians often complain of *rasehn*, "my head" (often saying it burns); *yazorehnyal*, "spinning" (not a true vertigo); and *libehn*, "my heart" (usually indicating dyspepsia rather than a cardiac problem). Most Ethiopians have faith in traditional healers and procedures. In children, uvulectomy (to prevent presumed suffocation during pharyngitis in babies), the extraction of lower incisors (to prevent diarrhea), and the incision of eyelids (to prevent or cure conjunctivitis) are common. Circumcision is performed on almost all men and 90% of women. Ethiopians do bloodletting for *moygnbagegn*, a neurologic disease that includes fever and syncope. Chest pain is treated by cupping. Ethiopians often prefer injections to tablets. Bad news is usually given to families of patients and not the patients themselves. *Zar* is a form of spirit possession treated by a traditional healer negotiating with the alien spirit and giving gifts to the possessed patient.

Bewoket had been sick for five or six years. He had been treated with traditional medicine and then was hospitalized a few times in Gojjam. His family finally took him home to die. That's when he ran away and headed for Addis.

Rick looked at the boy as he struggled to breathe and found it hard to believe that anyone who could barely sit up in bed could have walked three hundred kilometers to the capital. He examined Bewoket and concluded that the boy was being given the wrong drugs at the wrong doses, and they were being administered incorrectly. He decided to use this case as a teaching moment, though he had to be careful not to step on the sensitive toes of the medical staff.

Rick explained to his colleague that patients like Bewoket fail to absorb medication adequately so it is necessary to inject it directly into the vein. Bewoket needed Lasix, a diuretic, to clear fluid from his body, but the doctors in the hospital were afraid of overdosing him and had been keeping him on a low dose of oral Lasix. He had severe edema as fluid had built up throughout his system. "He needs to be peeing like a racehorse," Rick explained, "but now he's so overloaded with fluid that he has to sit bolt upright in bed just to breathe." Rick reflected on how much the boy had suffered coming alone to Addis Ababa, only to suffer more inside the hospital.

Rick then began a kind of Socratic exchange with the medical staff and went over the drugs that had been ordered—Lasix, quinidine, digoxin—how they should be administered, how to enhance their absorption, and how to prevent toxicity.

"Doctor," the nurse said, "why don't you send him to America for surgery?"

"It's far too late," Rick said. "His heart has so much damage at this point that he would be at extremely high risk for surgery. If he did survive, he'd still have a very limited life span. The only thing that would help him at this point is a transplant, and that's impossible. He's not American and he has no money. We have to be realistic. In the best case, he'll be stabilized, discharged, and live for a couple of years. Worst case: he'll die very soon."

As Rick got to know Bewoket over the coming days, he got a fuller story from the boy who had been so determined to get to Addis. His parents named him Bewoket, which means "by the will of God," and they came to believe that only God could keep him alive. Bewoket ran away from his home in the countryside when he overheard his father tell his mother that their son would

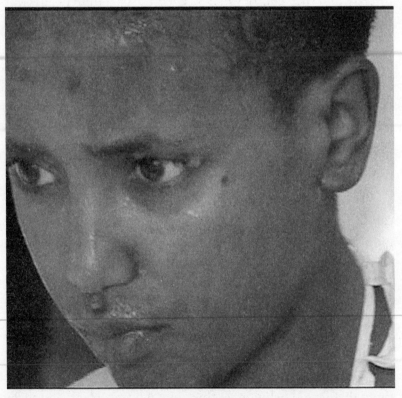

When Rick came upon Bewoket at the main hospital of Addis Ababa, the boy was struggling to breathe and fighting for his life.

be better off dead. He was too young to understand that his parents were only expressing the hope that his suffering would end, but the words terrified the boy and he bolted. He told Rick he started picking up food that had been discarded along the road and sold it to passersby to collect enough money to get to the capital. It took him two months to save 16 birr (about $2.50).

He paid 2 birr to ride on the top of a truck for the two-hour drive to the bus station in Debre Markos. There he hit a new obstacle: the ten-hour bus ride to Addis Ababa would cost 18 birr and he was 4 birr short. He was so close to his destination, but so far. It could take him weeks to scrounge up that kind of money. But he looked so weak and bedraggled that a kind soul at the bus depot took pity on him and agreed to sell him a ticket for the 14 birr he had in his pocket. So the story that he'd walked the entire distance turned out to be a bit of an exaggeration, although he had walked and hitchhiked for two days without any food. One night he slept on the dirt floor of a "hotel" room that cost him his last half birr (7 cents).

He arrived in Addis Ababa penniless, a complete stranger knowing no one. A traveler at the bus station saw that he was in distress and took him to Black Lion Hospital. There, his condition was noted as critical.

Black Lion is the main teaching hospital of Addis Ababa University. It is long past its prime. Rick said, "It was built in the 1970s by the Swiss, and run for the first couple of years as a Swiss hospital, with cleanliness and efficiency, piped-in oxygen to each bed and European nursing supervisors. Patients were issued plastic cards when they registered, and were able to get x-rays and arteriograms without difficulty."

The hospital was originally named Prince Makonnen, Duke

of Harrar Hospital, in memory of the son of Emperor Haile Selassie who died in an automobile accident.

"After Haile Selassie was overthrown," Rick says, "all references to his ubiquitous presence were destroyed, and the name was changed to Tikur Anbessa Hospital, or Black Lion. The Lion is one of the symbols of Ethiopia (and in fact, Haile Selassie referred to himself as Yehuda Anbessa, the Lion of Judah), and the Black Lions were a band of Ethiopians who fought the Italians during their occupation of the country in the late 1930s. Ethiopians now have made an Amharic pun out of the name, removing the *n* in Anbessa and, changing it to Tikur Abessa, or the Black Disaster.

"Physically it is falling apart. It is dirty, has leaking ceilings, broken windows, and smells like hell. The walls are covered with water stains, the paint is peeling, and the floor tiles are often missing. The piped-in oxygen died years ago. Some faucets have not worked for years, others run permanently. At times the entire building has no water. In fact, during the cholera epidemic that hit Addis Ababa in the mid-1980s, there were times that the only water in the neighborhood was in the fountains in front of the hospital, built by the North Koreans for the tenth anniversary of dictator Mengistu Haile Mariam's revolution.

"There's a critical shortage of supplies in all the hospitals here. . . . Last week, I dropped off a pregnant woman in labor to a city hospital. After twenty-four hours, they decided to do a cesarean section and called me at my office. 'This is an emergency,' they said, 'we need to operate. Bring us two pairs of sterile gloves, two bags of normal saline, one vial of ampicillin, and a sterile syringe and needle.' I immediately dispatched my nurse, delivered the supplies, and the patient was operated on successfully.

"At the same time, a heart patient I treat came up to Addis Ababa from Sidamo (in the southern part of the country) for some blood tests. He went to Black Lion Hospital and then returned back to me, asking for a syringe and needle so they could draw his blood.

"Recently the Finnish government paid more than half a million dollars to finance a study on restoration of the hospital. Their consultants estimated that it would cost about 200 million Ethiopian birr (about 32 million dollars) to renovate. The Ministry of Health pointed out that this sum was out of the question; it was virtually the entire health budget of the country, so last week the Finnish advisors simply packed up and went home."

This was the condition of the hospital that Bewoket had struggled so hard to reach. A few days after he met Bewoket, Rick could see that the boy's condition had worsened. He was not eating, was coughing up blood, a sign of fluid in the lungs, and his breathing had become more rapid. Rick was afraid the boy might not live through the night.

Rick decided that intravenous Lasix was now needed immediately to release the fluid in the boy's body and lungs, but there was none available at the hospital. He ran to his car and drove to the International Medicine Shop, where he bought ten vials of Lasix and prescribed an amount that the doctor on duty questioned but still administered in accordance with Rick's order.

Rick paid $10 for the Lasix. It probably saved Bewoket's life.

The new medications were a turning point, and every day the boy was a little better. But still he was as weak as a kitten and needed nourishment.

"I visited him daily," Rick remembers. "This was the high point of the day, not only for him but for others in the room as well. I would ask about his health and then always do something to try to make him laugh and lift his spirits. Each time I walked in, someone would say in a loud voice, 'Bewoket, your father is here.'"

The idea of being anyone's father was the furthest thing from Rick's mind. He took the remark "simply as a statement that I'm the one taking care of him." He added, "Now that I think of it, it's a lot easier being a doctor to a sick kid than a father to a sick kid."

WHILE RICK WAS STRUGGLING TO SAVE BEWOKET, a civil war three countries south of Ethiopia was convulsing in a genocidal tribal massacre that sent almost a million refugees spilling over the borders of Rwanda. Bewoket was still in a precarious state when Rick was suddenly dispatched to Goma, the decaying resort town on the border of Rwanda and Zaire (now the Democratic Republic of Congo), where the refugees were washing up on the shores of Lake Kivu, drinking the fetid water, contracting cholera, and dying by the thousands. When they started fleeing Rwanda in 1994, the JDC instructed Rick to put together a team to go immediately to the refugee encampment in Goma, Zaire, to provide emergency medical care.

Rick hired the first four Ethiopians who came in the door with passports, three of whom had never been out of the country and a fourth who had never been on an airplane. When Rick settled him into his seat, the man turned to him nervously. "Now, Rick, where is the parachute?" As they sped down the runway,

Rick watched as the man grabbed the armrests and repeated to himself, "We are going, we are going."

In Entebbe, the transfer point, they ran into lengthy delays and a horde of civil servants looking for bribes. Rick pleaded with the authorities. "I pointed out that refugees were dying in Zaire" and that "every hour earlier that we arrive, several lives will be saved." His appeal had no effect, and the transfer process continued at a glacial pace. While they waited, they passed the night on the concrete floor of a hangar along with several hundred American GIs who were part of a humanitarian rescue team.

When Rick awoke, he wanted to say his morning prayers. "It's a bit difficult to find a minyan in Entebbe these days," he noted dryly. So he found a corner of a nearby hangar and stood between some aging Russian MIGs, put on his tallith and tefillin, and performed the morning service alone.

Rick often turns to Hebrew texts and teachings for guidance on moral and ethical issues, so before he left Addis, he called the rabbi he had studied with in Maryland to seek his advice for the task of treating the sick and dying on the Rwandan border.

Rick explained: "I wondered if I should give priority to children (the future of the country), or perhaps to parents (if they died, their children would become orphans). Should I give each person fifteen minutes of time? Should I ignore the elderly or people who would take a long time to save? The rabbi's reply: I should not decide who to treat and who not to treat. Every life is precious. I should take critically ill patients in the order they come to me, and, once I start with such a patient, I must not interrupt their care unless it is medically appropriate."

When the JDC team finally reached the Kibumba refugee compound in Goma, they were confronted with an overwhelming horror, which Rick some months later attempted to describe in a letter to a colleague:

1 September, 1995
Hi Robert,
Seeing the camp for the first time is like
describing the Grand Canyon. Words could not
prepare me for it, even after working in Africa
for more than seven years. "Imagine a Woodstock
that goes on for miles," I faxed back to my office,
"hundreds of thousands of refugees living 20 miles
from any source of water. . . ." The lucky ones
had makeshift, waist-high, A-shaped homes, a
frame of twigs covered with blue plastic sheeting.
Others were simply lying in a ditch. The stench
of diarrhea was pervasive. Several dead bodies in
various stages of decay were lying nearby, maggots
swarming over them. The people appeared to be in
shock. Few moved. Few spoke. No smiles, nobody
crying. Children sat silently. Within a minute, I was
surrounded by potential patients. I saw a person
lying on his back with a piece of cloth over his face.
He was not moving. I picked up the handkerchief
to see his face. Perhaps 35 years old, thin, actually
emaciated, dehydrated. He was dead. "Next," I said.
I saw a person a few meters away lying in
watery excrement. I walked over and grabbed her
wrist. Feeble pulse, very rapid. . . . I started an

IV. . . . I went from patient to patient, hut to hut,
running back and forth seeing new patients and
changing bottles of IV fluid on previous ones. . . .
    At the end of the day, we would end up 100
meters from where we started, but during that
period of time, we would have each saved five or
ten or twenty lives, people who would otherwise
have died. It was certainly a drop in the vast ocean
of refugees, but I recalled that the Talmud says
"to save one life is to save an entire universe." I
faxed back to my office in New York that because
the five of us had come down to Zaire, 500–1000
refugees would be alive in the next couple of
weeks.

All my best,
Rick

The number of refugees suffering from cholera and assorted other deadly diseases kept growing. Rick interrupted his daily routine only long enough to put together local teams of translators and medics. Then, day after day, he made his way through the ever-expanding sea of refugees, distributing medicines and initiating intravenous hydration. At one point he wrote to the JDC that his work was slow and he didn't feel he was making much headway, but as he moved forward, he noticed that the people behind him were standing up.

This mass refugee migration had been touched off in April 1994 when the private plane carrying the presidents of Rwanda and Burundi was shot down by rocket fire. To this day it is not clear whether the assassinations were the work of a Tutsi-led rebel group or extremist Hutus. They each blame the other. But just as the assassination of the Archduke at Sarajevo touched off World War I, this incident became the spark that exploded long-held sectarian animosities into an episode of genocide in which the Hutu majority did their best to kill the Tutsi minority.

Detailed hit lists had been drawn up well in advance, part of a decades-long pattern of intertribal enmity. All those involved in the massacres were Rwandans, all were of the same ethnic origin, all spoke the same language; they had lived more or less together and went to the same churches, most of them Roman Catholic, a religion brought to them in the early part of the twentieth century by Belgian colonists. Many intermarried with each other.

Estimates of the numbers killed go up to one million. Most of the killings were carried out by very low-tech methods: people were slashed by machetes or beaten to death by clubs studded with nails.

"It is shocking to realize that it takes one person several minutes to kill another this way, if not longer, because people fight back," Rick said. "Often it will take several people several minutes to kill one individual, compounding the horror."

In some regions, 85 percent of the Tutsis were murdered, and, according to a report from the United Nations, 20 to 50 percent of Hutus (especially males) participated in the killings.

It was the direct involvement of the churches that Rick found the most shocking. "In the past, churches had been recognized as sanctuaries," he recalled. "This was no longer the case. In fact, many in the Catholic Church encouraged the carnage. A bishop got on the radio and announced 'The Tutsi graves are not full enough yet,' and in a mixed Hutu-Tutsi religious order, the Hutus killed the Tutsis. Many priests participated as well.

"The Rwandan Patriotic Army, largely Tutsi, eventually marched in, and the Hutus fled en masse to Zaire."

Meanwhile, the million or more refugees crowded along the border left women and children living side by side with the perpetrators of the genocide, the very same murderers who were responsible for the bloodbath within Rwanda. Many of those who had initiated the horrendous killings had themselves escaped over the border in search of food and medical care. They brought their weapons with them and, while seeking safe haven, they were also able to reconstitute their forces to fight another day. The uncomfortable fact was that if the humanitarian effort were to succeed in preventing epidemics and widespread starvation, there could be no discrimination between the murderers and their victims.

"These were very volatile people," Rick said of some of the refugees in the encampment. "Many of them had blood on their hands. It seemed that many of the men had the mentality of eight-year-olds, although with the ability to carry out their ideas, so if something bothered them they would simply threaten people with grenades.

"Several people were clubbed to death just 100 meters from our hospital because they were believed to be Tutsis. This was rather disheartening for those of us who simply wanted to save lives and not get involved in the ethnic dimension of the conflict. 'Why are we helping these people?' more than one person asked."

A friend asked Rick something that went to the heart of the refugee effort, the kind of question that is frequently asked: "Rick," he said, "after everything that has happened to the Jewish people, how can they give money to help the Hutus?"

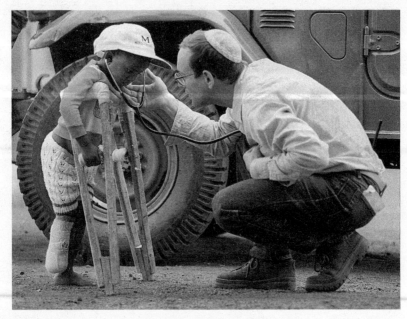

Rick trying to cheer up a small child whose lower leg was amputated.

"You can't sit by when people are dying like flies of cholera," he replied. He said that most of the people they were dealing with were women and children, but he said, "I was haunted by a bit of truth in what he said as well."

Rick recalled that a Mishna in *Pirke Avot,* a compilation of Hebrew ethical and moral principles, says, "The world depends on three things—on Torah study, on the service (of God), and on acts of kindness (Avot 1:2). These refugees are simple people, Christians and Moslems, risking their lives to escape the violence in their country. There is no obvious connection between the American Jewish community and these refugees, and assisting them is truly an act of kindness."

Some time later, Rick gave a speech in Rwanda where the JDC was funding a new back-to-school project for children of the genocide in which he explained—to himself as much as to his audience—why the Jews were helping in Rwanda.

> First of all, we want to help anywhere where human beings are suffering. Because of our own history, Jews are very sensitive to the suffering of others.
>
> Second, 50 years ago, we had our own Holocaust, the genocide organized by Adolf Hitler. During that period of time, many of us had nowhere to go, nowhere to escape to. The world hid its face from our suffering, and a total of six million people, one-third of all the Jews, were killed.
>
> This event, this genocide, has had a profound effect on us, and in some sense, all Jews today are somehow survivors of this.
>
> In Rwanda as well, you underwent a similar experience in many ways, and many Rwandans today are survivors as well.
>
> Thus we have great similarities in our histories and this too brings us together.

The refugee camp in Goma was, from the start, a study in shortages: nonexistent sanitation and inadequate supplies of food, firewood, medicines, and plastic sheeting, which had come to be valued almost more than human life. Around 60 percent of the refugees had no sheeting for their roofs.

"People seen walking with plastic sheets were frequently attacked," he said.

On a typical day at the camp, Rick and his staff woke up around 6:30 A.M., took bucket showers in outdoor stalls (only oc-

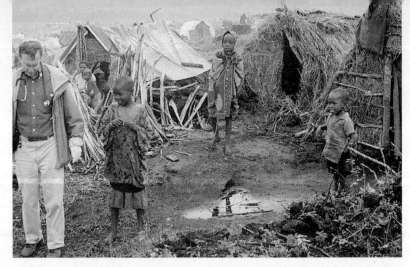

In Goma, the plastic sheeting used for roofs became worth more than human life.

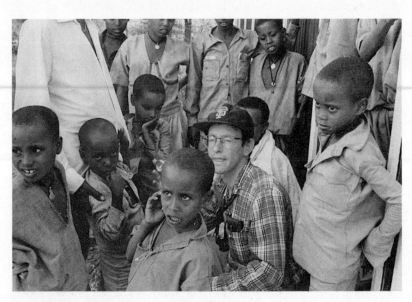

Rick with Goma refugees.

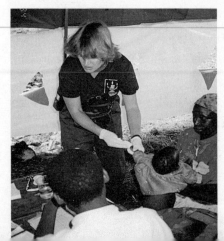

Nancy Larson treating a Rwandan refugee in Goma.

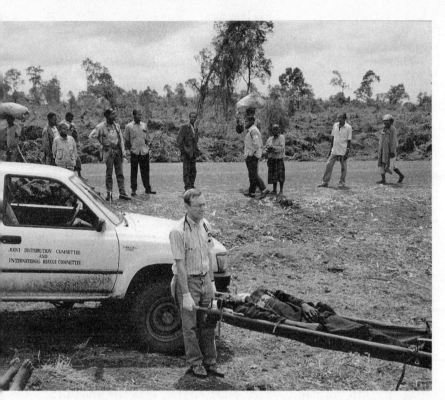

Rick in Goma.

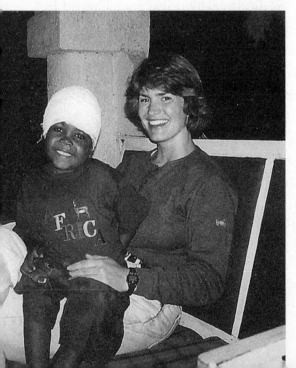

Taka after his surgery, with Nancy Larson, who said that after working all day with thousands of refugees, seeing this little guy struggling with his injuries brought the entire experience down to a level that was so real.

casionally with hot water), downed a cup or two of instant coffee and a bowl of cereal, and then headed off to do their work.

Until the United Nations organized a water operation (at a cost of $50,000 a day), Rick and his team filled their jerricans each morning from the San Francisco Fire Department's lakeside operation, added oral rehydration salts, and transported the cans on rented flatbed trucks through twenty miles of lush, green volcanic land to the camp.

This was always a perilous trip, impeded by the thousands of people living along the roadside and children everywhere who would jump on any moving vehicle. Rick said it took good drivers, which meant Western drivers, and big sticks to chase away the kids. In fact, he said, Médecins Sans Frontières (Doctors Without Borders) actually had a budget line for "child beaters."

"The British, who took over from them, considered the language too inflammatory," Rick said, "so they kept the line in the budget but changed the description to the more benign 'crowd control.'"

The severity of the medical problems was compounded by the difficulty of coordinating with the other aid groups from around the world, the red tape to import needed equipment and medicine, and the never-ending bribery that was required to navigate what Rick called the "kleptocracy" of Zaire in order to obtain the wherewithal to carry on their work.

Just registering the refugees was a multi-stage adventure. First, people were given wristbands and then registered several days later. But within hours, the wristbands, which were a passport to food and medical care, were being sold in the local market. There were all sorts of tricks. A refugee who had been given a wristband would slide it up his arm, get rebanded and sell the extras. Some people kidnapped local children and registered them as refugees to get extra food rations. Others used bleach to wash off the gentian violet that was stamped on their arms to indicate registration; then they reapplied, were reregistered, and got double rations.

"One of the ironies of refugee situations," Rick said, "is that the refugees get far more attention and far better care than the locals who live in similar circumstances nearby."

Rick created a manual for the treatment of common ailments, and a nurse came from New Orleans to train a group of health aides. She selected forty people and taught them how to take a census and how to identify malnutrition, dehydration, fever, and diarrhea. With Rick's manual and her training, they were sent out into the field to find sick people.

"We divided our sector into thirteen segments," Rick said, "and painted numbers on all the homes, registered each family, and gave them health cards with their house numbers on them."

Rick considered himself fortunate to get the help of two extraordinary American paramedics who wanted to volunteer to work in the Rwandan crisis and had faxed their résumés to a number of humanitarian organizations. These women, Nancy Larson and Debbie Fisher, had been rejected by Pat Robertson's Operation Blessing after they failed to give an appropriate answer to this question: "Describe your relationship with Jesus." The JDC was happy to recruit them.

Rick described Nancy as "a thirtyish paramedic from Minneapolis who grew up as one of nine children on a hog farm in Minnesota." She had been working with Debbie for years on the streets of Minneapolis, where they had become known affection-ately as "the harlots from hell." (Nancy says she didn't know the meaning of the word *harlot*.) Nancy also worked as a paramedic on an FBI SWAT team covering a number of midwestern states and just missed being sent to the confrontation in Waco, Texas. Rick said she was naturally enthusiastic and well organized; in addition to all her nursing work, she took over the distribution of the precious plastic sheeting and monitored the medical team's own security. She also took charge of a little boy named Taka, a five-year-old left for dead in a ditch.

He came into their lives one day when Rick was driving down a road in a pickup truck filled with his staff. Some ref-ugees on the side of the road signaled him to slow down and handed up the dying boy, who had been severely beaten in the head. Taka had been separated from his mother months before while they were crisscrossing Rwanda looking for refuge from the genocide. He had been searching for her ever since. All he remembered was that she was wearing a red blouse.

Rick took the boy to the Israeli field hospital, where he under-went a series of delicate operations, and when the Israelis closed down their clinic, Taka came to stay in Rick's, and sometimes in Nancy's, tent. When they went into the refugee camps each day, Taka hung out with the mechanics and the cooks and anybody who wouldn't shoo him away. He managed to charm the entire contingent, but when Rick was around, Taka stuck to his leg as if attached by a bungee cord, as Nancy tells it.

After traveling all across Rwanda on foot for three months to get to safety, Taka was never sure where his next meal was coming from, so he started pilfering food, stockpiling it under his pillow for a rainy day. Then he started to gorge himself to the point that they had to protect him from himself and actually hired a nanny to control him while Rick and Nancy and the others were out in the field working with the refugees.

"Taka became the center of our lives there," Nancy remembered. "To see hundreds of thousands of people suffering in the camps every day was overwhelming and then to come home and have this little guy full of life struggling with this injury, that brought the whole experience down to a level that was so real."

In time, Nancy was able to piece together Taka's story. He remembered that the family was on a hillside digging up manioc when a neighbor screamed that soldiers were coming and they needed to flee. Following his mother, who carried a baby, and his stepfather, who carried another child, Taka tried to keep up as the family found their way first to the Tanzanian border, which was closed when they got there, and then toward the Zaire border, which they reached after three months. During the trek there was a firefight, and Taka was separated from the family. He survived on his own for a month, turning up rocks to eat the worms and grubs he found underneath. Some nights he would sneak over to campfires to warm himself, and occasionally he would climb under a blanket where a fellow refugee was sleeping and would awake in the morning to find a toddler sharing his bunk. Eventually two women, moved by his lonely plight, told him he could walk with them.

When he got to the border, Taka told Nancy that there were men checking people's identity cards. He said soldiers were separating the refugees, apparently Tutsi from Hutu, according to what was written on what he called their "credit cards." On one side, as he tells it, he saw soldiers holding guns to the heads or stomachs of the people in that line. Then, in Taka's words, "they'd lie down on the ground and go to sleep."

One of the women told him he'd better make a run for it because he didn't have his credit card. That's when he got smashed in the head with the machete.

AFTER TREATMENT AT THE ISRAELI field hospital and being coddled at the volunteers' camp, Taka was finally sent to New York University for further surgery. The doctor, who was thinking of adopting him himself, took him to Minneapolis for a visit, where Taka met Nancy's husband, Kyle, a police officer. "Taka went crazy for this six foot four cop," Nancy says, describing her husband. He announced to the doctor, "I'm going to stay here. I like it here." Four years and a lot of paperwork later, Taka was formally adopted; Nancy thinks he may be the only Rwandan child of the genocide legally adopted in America. He's fallen into a suburban family that represents the best America has to offer, with devoted, hardworking parents who envelop him in love, with Debbie as his godmother and a network of doctors and nurses from around the country who met him in Goma and keep abreast of his progress.

Kyle's most treasured memory of Taka as a child was of the time he took him to his first baseball game, the Minnesota Twins, of course:

> He's fresh out of Rwanda, five or six years old, nobody
> sitting around us, and I'm pointing things out to him

and explaining the game. Then someone takes the seat next to us and I turn to my right. There is this mountain of a guy with broad shoulders, huge biceps bulging out of his white T-shirt.

This was the year that *The Lion King* movie came out and we had watched it over and over again. There's a scene with the warthog that clearly made an impression on Taka, and so he turns to this big guy and says, "Hi, Mr. Pig." I thought, *Oh boy, this is gonna hurt when this guy slugs me.* But the guy says to him, "What's your name?" "I'm Taka Larson," he replies in his high little voice. So the big guy says to this small black boy, "Larson, eh, are you Norwegian?" And he turns to me and says, "Dad, am I Norwegian?"

Taka became an avid hockey player in high school and attended Southwest Minnesota State University before transferring to the University of Minnesota, Duluth. He has become a young man with a powerfully strong physique. When Rick visits, he and Taka compare muscles, and Rick shows off his wrestling stance, a reminder of the days in Goma when Jesse Ventura provided some laughs when they were needed.

Rick, it seems, was an All-Star Wrestling fan and knew all the names, all the teams, and all the wrestling moves. Nancy remembers that Rick couldn't get over the fact that Minnesota had actually elected an All-Star wrestler, Jesse Ventura, as governor. He kept saying, "You can't make this up." Nancy noticed that whenever Rick sensed the tension building among the staff he would resort to the nuttiness of the wrestling world to lighten the atmosphere. "His crazy antics helped you forget about the horrible things going on around you and provided a really good belly laugh," Nancy said.

Ventura's nickname was "Jesse the Body." For comic relief, Nancy and Debbie came up with "Rick the Body Hodes," which they considered hilariously incongruous for the pint-sized Jewish doctor living in Africa.

THE REFUGEES IN THE CAMP had organized themselves according to their villages. They began each day with a search for food—distributed when available by the World Food Organization—water, medical care, and firewood.

"You can imagine the ecological damage caused by 200,000 people crossing the road into the Zairian National Park to cut firewood," Rick wrote in September 1995. "The forest, previously near the roadside, was moving further and further back every week. European technical experts calculated that there would have to be 200 truckloads of wood delivered daily to the camp to avoid this deforestation."

Aid groups from around the world responded to the crisis—Rick called them an alphabet soup of nongovernmental organizations, like CARE, as well as the United States Army, the San Francisco Fire Department, Save the Children, Feed the Hungry, an Israeli team, and Pat Robertson's Operation Blessing, which drew Rick's vigorous scorn.

Rick said the Robertson group arrived and announced that things were not being done well and that they would be happy to take over.

"They had no logistical support, had not practiced African medicine, and were lost in Goma," he recalled. "They set up two small tents (similar to the ones I slept in outside in my backyard when I was nine years old) with a huge professional sign: 'Operation Blessing: Medical Strike Force.'" Rick's team started asking him why they didn't have a sign.

Rick quickly realized that Operation Blessing's main agenda was not so much to save the lives of the refugees as to save their souls by converting them to evangelical Protestantism.

"They would approach people who had no plastic sheeting and ask them to pray to Jesus for sheeting," he said. "A week later, they would deliver the sheeting, a sure sign that the prayers had been answered." What's more, he said, they reported this miracle openly at an NGO coordinating meeting.

But he also learned—from government officials as well as from newspaper and magazine reports—that while medicine took second place to their evangelism, there was a third item on their agenda that took precedence over the other two.

"Why," he asked, "did this tiny NGO have three Canadian Caribou twin-engine airplanes flying around? And why did they have a large office in Kinshasa, with state-of-the-art communications equipment and ex-U.S. Navy (born-again Christian) Special Forces as security people?" The answer, Rick discovered, was what he called, "a girl's best friend"—*DIAMONDS*.

Officials told Rick that Robertson had struck a deal with Mobutu to prospect for alluvial diamonds in several Zaire riverbeds, and the planes were used to fly in diamond dredging equipment. The pilots themselves later publicly accused Robertson of diverting the planes from their humanitarian mission, a violation of the organization's tax-exempt status.

As new waves of refugees arrived, the different aid groups started tripping over each other. Some were exceedingly effective, others were not. Rick called CARE-Deutschland "one of the biggest jokes in Goma." They arrived well equipped with two hundred volunteers, including doctors, nurses, and do-gooders, and, as Rick told it, "twenty shiny new Land Rover ambulances, high-tech satellite phones and fax machines, an array of (sometimes inappropriate) drugs chosen by a committee in Germany, including cyclophosphamide [for cancer] and acyclovir [for herpes viruses], and a budget of millions. We're talking deep pockets. So what could go wrong?" What, indeed. Rick says they hadn't a clue and ran around like the Keystone Kops. They rotated staff every two weeks, had nowhere to live, and had no experience with African illnesses.

"CARE was hit with terrible publicity in Germany dealing with their lack of organization and their poor planning," Rick said.

They were so inefficient, in fact, that the word in the field was that they weren't really Germans but Italians speaking German! After some weeks, however, Rick said they found their footing and with the help of an experienced coordinator, made a contribution. Rick also volunteered to help the German team. He observed, "I started going to their compound every week or two and gave a seminar for a couple of hours on refugee medicine, going through cholera, measles, meningitis, shigella, and malaria; use of drugs, triage, public health measures, and vitamin A; and answering as many questions as possible. (There is something a bit ironic about a short Jewish guy with a *kippa,* lecturing in front of two hundred Germans.)"

The camp presented Rick with a tableau of human folly. He

was struck, for example, by the visit of a congressional delegation from the United States: "They ventured only a few meters into the camp for a photo opportunity surrounded by their aides, then turned to their photographers and asked, 'You sure you got this on film, guys?' One congressman who stepped in shit spent ten minutes wiping his shoes. (In contrast, it seemed that we were stepping in shit every ten minutes.)"

The camps went through waves of disease. First there was cholera, and once that dissipated, shigella dysentery (a highly contagious bacterial infection causing severe cramps, vomiting, fever, and explosive bloody diarrhea), followed by malaria and then measles and meningitis. Several aid groups started immunizations against measles and meningitis and gave the children biscuits as a reward for accepting the injection. Many children got multiple shots just so they could get more biscuits. The immunizations lessened the incidence of disease, but when new refugees came to the camps, they brought new rounds of disease.

Rick was frequently asked if the aid that was contributed really reaches the people. "Well," he would usually reply, "most of it." But he said there was plenty of fraud: "We had drugs stolen, plenty of cement (used for permanent latrines) taken, a generator walked out of the hospital compound one Sunday afternoon, and even a donated vehicle disappeared. . . . In the camp things like cameras and jackets would disappear if you turned your head for a second. MSF had six tons of food stolen in one night. One morning a night nurse was found taking home the drugs she was supposed to have administered on her shift."

There was no shortage of local workers, all of them representing themselves as being fully qualified. But among the many job seekers, Rick found drivers who'd never sat in the front seat of a car, nurses who'd never taken a pulse, and doctors who did not know which side of the body the liver was on or where to find the spleen. Rick was sure that if he'd requested 747 pilots he would have had fifty applicants the next day. There was competition among the aid groups for well-trained staff, and the locals became adept at playing one group against the other. But Rick explained that it is unethical to hire away an NGO worker for a higher salary, and finally, after a long series of meetings, the various groups agreed to a universal pay scale.

Once hired, the locals demanded payment in dollars because the local currency was virtually worthless and continued to lose value by the day. Besides, there were no banks in Goma. NGOs would take money from their accounts with Western banks in Nairobi and fly in sums like $20,000 or $50,000 in brown paper bags every week or two to pay their local staff. Here's how it worked, according to Rick. They would radio a message to Nairobi saying, "We need reading material, send in twenty comic books," and $20,000 would be hand-carried in on the next flight.

Rick said salaries for local workers went from around $1.50 per day for a cleaner to $8 for a doctor. "There were a couple of ways to pay people," he said. "If enough small bills were not available to pay in dollars someone could go to one of the street corners . . . where the black marketeers hang out and return with boxes and boxes of local currency, known in short as Z's. It would take two full-time counters three days to count out the biweekly salary for the IRC's local staff. They would scream for days if they were paid in local currency. I don't blame them, but we often had no other choice."

Dealing with the health emergency was almost easier than dealing with the local government bureaucracy. At every turn Rick was reminded that Zaire ran on bribes and extortion, a country, he said, "where President Mobutu is worth billions and charters the Concorde when he flies to Europe, but where the army, civil servants, and diplomats have not been paid in several years."

In Goma, policemen would stand on the roadside looking for people they could extort money from. Rick said, "'You did not put on your turn signal,' one would say, 'pay me ten dollars.' They would demand documentation, and even though this may be complete (driver's license, registration, etc.), it was never enough. 'You don't have your baptism certificate,' one would say. 'Ten dollars.' Sometimes they were completely honest. At the airport, one said to me, 'Please give me some money. I am very thirsty. I need some beer.'

"They invented taxes left and right. NGO vehicles carried their NGO flag and had prominent stickers on the sides. This was an opportunity for a fine: advertising tax. And one of our male workers was fined ten dollars for wearing an earring."

Rick called the airport "a gold mine for Zairian civil servants to be posted: those in charge of it have a virtual looting franchise." He said, "During the initial phase of the emergency, truckloads of relief supplies drove away never to be seen again. The soldier at the airport with the key to the men's room wanted to charge me 1,000 Z's (about a quarter) to pee there; instead I went to the side of the runway like every other Zairian and added my nitrogen to their soil."

He said, "We became adept at dealing with these people. At the airport, where it was almost routine for authorities to confiscate someone's passport or radio or ID on trumped-up charges (such as being a Ugandan spy or not having registered properly), we paid one of the senior people a $10 'no problems' fee every time one of our planes landed. Our problems decreased by 90 percent. And after we gave the brother of one of the border guards a job, it became much easier for us to cross over into Rwanda."

Outside the airport there was still another regime to be greased. Rick recalled: "Our rented bus filled with hospital staff was stopped one morning in front of the airport and the driver's papers checked. . . . Several of us got out as well to watch what was happening and to radio our base to let them know why we would be late getting back. The Zairian soldier looked up with amusement. 'Go ahead, use your radios,' he said. 'Call whoever you want. Call Mobutu and tell him he hasn't paid me for three years!' He finally confiscated the driver's papers and promised to give them back in return for several beers that evening."

One evening, frustrated with the callousness of the officials and overwhelmed by the sickness around him, Rick was exhausted. "What type of people go into this work?" he wondered out loud. He turned to Barb Smith, a nurse with a Ph.D. in psychology who had done volunteer work off and on for years, and asked her.

"There is no one type," she replied. "In the end you just have to want to do it."

Rick was dissatisfied with her answer, but months later he decided she was probably correct.

"Rick, face it," a friend said recently, "none of us is normal; otherwise we'd be back in regular jobs having regular lives. Look at the people who do this: great egotists, lone rangers, people out to save the world, born-again Christians dedicated to spreading the good word, people who are running from God knows what, do-gooders, and people who are just a bit off and who need more space."

Rick put it another way in a letter to a friend. "Let me point out that all of us out here are a bit crazy; normal doctors don't end up in the third world for years on end." But he said he had developed a pretty clear understanding of what it takes to be a success in what he called this refugee business.

"Flexibility," he wrote,

> *the ability to talk with and work with other people, the ability to not sulk when one's ideas are not accepted, and to keep common goals in mind; a bit of looseness and humor always help. Refugees rarely say thank you, so people who expect gratitude are soon disillusioned. Experience doesn't really count for too much as long as there are some experienced people you can learn from. I'd give it a 50 percent for flexibility, 50 percent for ability to work with others, and the other 50 percent for all other intangibles. (I realize that comes to more than 100 percent, but it's a big job.)*

How do we keep going, surrounded by death, and stay relatively sane? Rick would ask himself. "Part I is to stay very focused," he said. "I recall one day in early August when three young children we had worked on for hours the previous day died in the first hour. I sat down for a moment, put my head in my hands, and thought about this catastrophe. I realized that if I could not function well, people would die as a result. So I stood up and went back to work, focusing on my role, which was to rehydrate as many people as possible, and not to dwell on the extraordinary tragedies surrounding me. Part II is to get some rest and distance from time to time. We insisted that workers take one day off per week and a full week off for R & R in Nairobi every six or seven weeks."

In spite of this, he said, several people decompensated, used drugs or went on alcoholic binges, and had to be flown out. One French employee got drunk, wrecked a car, then took off his clothes and lay down on the living room couch. When someone suggested that he put some clothes on, he replied: "Leave me alone, it's my day off!"

5

ONE GOOD DEED LEADS TO ANOTHER

DURING THE ALMOST SIX MONTHS that Rick was away from Addis, Bewoket had been discharged from the hospital to Mother Teresa's mission, where he had a bed of his own in a spotless dormitory that he shared with thirty other kids. He had everything he needed, it would seem: companionship, his medicine, his food. But he was not eating and was very depressed.

"He told me he wanted to live at my house," Rick said.

Bewoket ran away from Mother Teresa's and Rick found him at the hospital. "I took him home and he slept on cushions on my living room floor," Rick said. "The following day I returned him to the mission but we cut a deal: once a week he could sleep at my home."

But he was soon back in the hospital again, this time with dysentery. Rick remembers discussing the case with the doctor on duty.

"This is a tough situation. On the one hand, he's sick as hell and dehydrated. On the other hand, too much fluid can push him over into pulmonary edema and kill him."

Nevertheless, Bewoket recovered enough to go back to the mission.

"This is a kid with more than nine lives and he made it through," Rick said.

But he was still seriously depressed and required a feeding tube; at the age of twelve or maybe thirteen, he weighed only fifty-three pounds.

"We are fighting for his life," one of the nuns told Rick. "You made a big mistake, Doctor. You attached yourself to him so much he won't live without you. You must do something."

Rick was not convinced he'd made a mistake, but he felt obligated to help. He recalled: "I violated the Sabbath rest by driving across town to pick up Bewoket. He was too weak to step up into my car, so I lifted him and placed him in the front seat. He spent the day at my house. As soon as he arrived, he was a different person, still incontinent and having dysentery, but he sat up, he ate, he smiled, he walked around a bit and played with my dogs. I told him that if he eats well on Sunday at the mission, he could spend Monday at my home."

Bewoket wanted to stay there permanently. "I had no interest in taking him in," Rick said. "I did, however, have great interest in keeping him alive."

The nurses at Mother Teresa's would call Rick every time Bewoket's condition took a new turn. After a while, Rick realized it would be more efficient to have the boy at home where he could see him every day and keep a running check on him and his medications.

"It was a lot easier than being called away every time a nurse was concerned about him," he said. "So I took him home and gave him a living room couch to sleep on," Rick said. "He was happy with this."

But Bewoket then developed active tuberculosis; he was emaciated and had an enlarged liver and a distended belly.

"I remember going to London and sitting in the British Medical Library trying to think about what might be done," Rick said. "I would pick up liver textbooks. And heart textbooks. It seemed that he had end-stage liver disease."

That turned out to be chronic hepatitis B, a disease for which there was no treatment at the time. Then by chance Rick noticed in a medical journal that a Harvard doctor had written a paper about the use of lamivudine, an AIDS drug, against chronic hepatitis B. The drug was not yet approved, but Rick thought it just might save Bewoket's life.

He returned to Addis and now had a very sick child living with him. "I would lie in bed and hear him coughing," he said. "It was haunting, really."

But Bewoket had a place to call home, and once he was there others followed. Rick's life was transformed as well. He started returning regularly to Mother Teresa's, treating anyone who came in the door.

"Somehow my world was changed by taking care of Bewoket," he marvels. In the Jewish tradition, it says *mitzvah goreret mitzvah,* which loosely translated means "one good deed leads to another." A mitzvah, he says, is not simply a good deed.

A mitzvah is a commandment from God that sets you on a certain trajectory.

"If you're doing good, you can't do evil," Rick says. "The Bewoket story set me on a new trajectory in which one thing led to another. I have a lot to thank Bewoket for."

What he could thank Bewoket for was work without end but also an opportunity to make a difference in the lives of many. He didn't realize it at the time, but Rick had found his true calling.

"What hope do these kids have?" he asks, contemplating their chances if he didn't try to help. "Very little at present. In this country where the health budget is about half a dollar per person, and the prospects for controlling the streptococcus (and many other diseases) are low, it is likely that things will continue as is, at least for the next decade or two. Economic development, medical education, and expanded primary health care may improve things after a while." But it will be a long time.

NOT LONG AFTER BEWOKET WAS SETTLED into his new home, Rick was sent to yet another refugee camp, this one in Kigoma on Lake Tanganyika in Tanzania. He had become the JDC's point man in Africa, and whenever something went wrong that they wanted to make right, Rick was the first line of defense, the first dispatched to the scene. When Dean Rusk was secretary of state for Presidents Kennedy and Johnson, he used to say that while Americans are asleep, two-thirds of the world is awake and committing some kind of outrage. Those outrages tended to explode most frequently in Rick's broadly defined neighborhood, which eventually stretched from Rwanda and Tanzania to Turkey and Kosovo. Whenever the call came in, Rick had to drop his day-to-day work of treating patients and enter a wider ocean where the medical problems were far more numerous and even more urgent.

But now Rick had a child at home. Bewoket was still frail and still in need of both nurturing and frequent medical attention. It was becoming clear that his damaged heart would soon need surgery. Fortunately, when Rick was in Goma the year before, he had asked Endale, an older former patient, to move in to oversee the house; now he would also take care of Bewoket while he was away.

Kigoma in 1996 presented many of the same miseries as and the same catastrophes of Goma, but this time most of the refugees made their way from Zaire instead of Rwanda. They would pay what they could afford—something like $15, four chickens, and a goat—to travel by boat across Lake Tanganyika from Zaire to reach the temporary refugee encampments in Tanzania. Each day the number of sick and dying there increased, with three hundred to a thousand souls coming and going in a camp crowded with ninety-two hundred very sick people on a site that could barely accommodate three thousand. Rick was the only medical doctor in the temporary camp, which made him responsible for all of them. At their peak, the camps along the border were overwhelmed with fifty thousand refugees struggling against the ravages of pneumonia, malaria, and cholera.

Every now and then, on days when he became especially discouraged, Rick daydreamed about a more simple life, painting houses, for example, as he had done in college. One day he was confronted with a thirty-five-year-old woman in her twelfth labor, pregnant with twins, and with two critically ill babies whom he had treated before. Both babies had high fevers, one of them gasping for breath with severe pneumonia. They looked terrible. Neither had improved on antibiotics.

He ordered more antibiotics for the two babies and took the pregnant woman to the maternity clinic. She made it to the hospital without delivering in the car, but an hour later, Rick got a radio call telling him both babies had died.

"I felt like I'd been shot in the heart," he said, and kept asking himself what he could have done differently.

One afternoon, when he'd gone to do rounds at the government hospital in Kigoma, Rick noticed that the sun was setting and turned to his translator. "Excuse me," he said, "I need five minutes for afternoon prayers." With that, he stepped into a corner of the open ward and, in view of the patients, prayed Mincha.

When someone tried to ask Rick a question, the translator stopped him.

"Wait," he said, "the doctor is praying."

"What country is he from?" a refugee asked after seeing Rick's *kippa*.

"He is an Israeli person, a Jew," the translator replied.

When he said his final amen, Rick turned to the translator and said, "Tell them I was praying for their health."

"I didn't know Israelis pray for non-Israeli people," the man replied.

"Of course we do," Rick said, smiling.

"I'll remember that," he answered.

Wryly noting that not many people in East Africa were cel-
ebrating Hanukah that December, Rick set aside a moment each
evening in his clinic to observe the holiday. Some of the refugees
had seen the menorah on his desk and had asked about it, so, as
the sun was setting, he called a few of them into his room, lit the
first of the candles, and told them the story of Hanukah and the
rededication of the Temple following the Maccabees' victory over
the forces of Antiochus IV. Some visitors from Amnesty International translated as he described the consecrated oil that was
sufficient for just one day but miraculously lasted for eight. He
also explained that Jews repeated the ceremony each year, as he
was here, to thank God for their freedom.

The refugees asked Rick what it meant to be Jewish.

"It was like being asked to teach the Torah while standing
on one foot," he said, wondering to himself how he could con-
dense a lifetime of religious study into an answer for these ear-
nest young men. He did not want to get into a debate, and in no
way did he want to be seen as proselytizing, so he said simply:
"The Jewish people were asked by God to be examples to the
world of three things: honesty, morality, and kindness. That is
the point."

With that brief and certainly inadequate answer, Rick went
back to work. The next day, as darkness fell, five young men
from the group of refugees asked to see him. They sat down on a
wooden bench in the clinic and were very serious and quiet, their
demeanor very much like the one they would adopt when they
were about to report a death.

One of them, who spoke some English, began the conversation nervously. "We want to speak with you," he said. As Rick

started to ask what he could do for them, the young man blurted out the reason for their coming into his office:

"We agree."

"Agree to what?" Rick asked, having no idea what they were talking about.

"We want to join the Jewish people," the young man replied.

"I almost fell off my chair in astonishment," Rick remembered, still amazed so many years later.

"We're not the only ones," the young man continued, "there are many others. We spoke with them. They also agree."

"How many?" Rick asked, now curious. "Maybe twenty," the young man replied.

Rick said, "I remember thinking that if I were a Mormon missionary, I would go to Mormon heaven immediately, without stopping on Go or collecting $200, but I have no intention of being a missionary for anything. They asked me to teach them something about my religion. At best, if I can add a bit to their awareness of God and increase their level of honesty or morality or spread a bit of kindness, that is plenty. But I don't want to do anything to encourage converts."

With that in mind, Rick turned to his prayer book, the siddur, and read from the Mishna from Pirkei Avot: "Consider three things and you will not come into the grip of sin: know what is above you—a watchful eye, an attentive ear, and all your deeds are recorded in a book." Then, he added, "The important thing is not to be a Jew. The important thing is to believe in God, to love him and fear him, to avoid bribery and slander, to be honest and upright and kind."

The point he was trying to make, he said, was that when we

behave correctly, right here, it brings us somehow close to God as well.

The young man then asked if they could join him the next night when he would again light the candles.

"If you like," Rick replied.

DURING THE TWO MONTHS RICK spent in Kigoma, the big event was to be a visit by the Tanzanian prime minister, who was coming to inspect the camps. Rick was told that he should be at his clinic when the entourage arrived.

"The prime minister and his motorcade of police cars and Land Rovers drove into the camp," he remembered. "They saw the rain, the mud, the crowds huddled in shelters and under the parapets, and simply turned around and drove off.

"People watched in amusement as the cars drove in and out again. If an American president did something like that, it would be a huge scandal. But here in Africa nobody expects well-dressed leaders to step into the mud to meet barefoot refugees, even when protected by twenty umbrellas."

A couple of times a day, when Rick too had to get away from the torrential rains, the constant barrage of patients, the radio calls, staff with questions, the mud, the noise, and the crowds and the crying babies and the multitude of smells drifting in through the window, he retreated into the supply closet, his makeshift sanctuary.

"Oh, the doctor's office in Africa," said a passerby who stuck his head in.

Rick would sit on an IV fluid box surrounded by drugs and

drinking water, write on his clipboard, and listen to his battery-powered shortwave radio, set to the BBC World Service.

In a journal he kept while he was in Tanzania, he wrote about this closet sanctuary:

> This is where I pray Mincha and Ma'ariv, drink water, and eat my peas or beans. I've been eating huge amounts of boiled beans or dried peas, my main staple here. One important thing here is not to become dehydrated. The best way I've found to do this is to drink normally throughout the day, then around 4 P.M. to drink as much as physically possible—often a liter or more. I repeat this a half hour later for a second time, and soon feel revived.

Amid all the crowding and the misery and the mud, Rick actually took a moment to write a thank-you note to his boss to tell him how much he appreciated the opportunity to take part in the refugee operation:

> *I like the challenges of working in different environments, trying to understand other cultures, pick up languages and figure out how things work. . . . I don't like being tied down to any one thing or place. There is great satisfaction at the end of the day knowing that I have saved several lives, satisfaction one doesn't get treating sinusitis in Rockville, Roslyn, or Rochester.*

Rick was thrilled and, he admits, even astonished when he returned to Addis to find that Bewoket had responded to the lamivudine and was on his way to being cured of hepatitis B. He was becoming stronger and his appetite had improved. "To my amazement his hepatitis B test became negative. This is quite rare—it happens about 1 percent of the time." With Bewoket's heart stable and his hepatitis B cured, Rick started to consider sending him for heart surgery in America.

Rick doesn't seem to dwell for long on the sheer pleasure of getting something right, but it is clear that his inner soul is nourished. I'm beginning to think it's addictive, this business of saving lives, and Rick seeks it out like a junkie seeks out a fix. How else can one explain why Rick returned time and time again to Mother Teresa's, where Bewoket had found shelter and where the need for his medical skills was unending?

Ethiopia, as Rick says, is a tough place to be sick and a tough place to be a doctor. The national health budget is barely enough for a single province. The Mengistu regime, taking a page from the Chinese and Cambodians, started sending intellectuals to the countryside for reeducation, creating a huge brain drain with doctors and medical students abandoning the country as quickly as they could. According to the latest figures available, from 2007, there are only 1,806 doctors in all of Ethiopia, but more than half of them have left the national health service for higher salaries with international organizations and NGOs. The remaining 939 are all that remain in the public sector for a population of eighty-two million. The government spent 15.5 birr—the equivalent of $1.50—per person on health care in 2007. Major drugs are unavailable, laboratories cannot do basic blood work, and the lack of sterile gloves can hold up a breast biopsy for a week. Abraham Verghese, an émigré doctor who started his medical studies in Addis and now teaches at Stanford, said, "The very thing that stopped me from staying are Rick's starting point—the lack of resources and the huge needs. Rick scratches and borrows and begs and gets what he needs."

According to a U.S. government report, Ethiopia is "in a downward spiral of hunger, poverty, and recurring food crises." Malnutrition and poverty are at 40 percent. Ethiopia is either the most populous or the second most populous country in Africa (statistics vary) and the poorest but one on the entire continent. It maintains the largest standing army on the continent, but its infrastructure is decayed and barely functional.

Whenever he had some free time, Rick would drive over to Mother Teresa's and walk through the series of large dormitories, each with thirty or forty beds right next to one another, all of them clean, crowded, and well tended. The patients were thin, often emaciated, perhaps 90 percent of them infected with HIV. The children had a variety of illnesses, some retarded, some with congenital deformities, others with acquired infections. There were about six hundred patients altogether, about the same number as the university hospital, but at Mother Teresa's, unlike the hospital, there were usually basic drugs and IV fluids for the patients. Rick volunteered to consult on the most difficult cases, and an international staff of nuns working quietly and efficiently eight to twelve hours each day provided care and medication.

One young nurse from Italy, who was particularly caring, caught Rick's eye. "I would daydream and wonder if she'd convert to Judaism," he recalled. "Fat chance. Once I invited her out for pizza. She smiled and told me they're not allowed to leave the mission."

—⊸∿⊷—

ON RETURNING HOME ONE DAY, Rick asked Bayelign, his house guard, what time it was. When he said he didn't know, Rick asked him to check. "I can't read or write, you know," he said. Rick first met Bayelign when he was working as a day laborer on a project near the JDC clinic. He invited the young man to join him at a kiosk to have juice, Rick's equivalent of the cocktail hour. When Bayelign told Rick of his life as a child soldier, Rick hired him on the spot to work for him and then to live in his house.

Bayelign is the oldest of Rick's ever-growing family, now a smiling, curly-haired giant of a man whose main goal in life these days is to join an uncle in Israel. The child of a Jewish father and a mother he believes was Jewish, he tells of observing Jewish holidays when he was growing up in Gondar; he dreams of serving in the Israeli Army in the tough Golani Brigade. He has had more than enough experience for that.

His father left home to fight in the Ethiopian army and never returned. His mother died when he was young, and, now a grown man, Bayelign still weeps when he speaks of her. After he was orphaned, he tried to join Mengistu's army because he was told that as a recruit he would be fed. But he was so undernourished, he couldn't pass the weight test, so at age thirteen he put on long pants for the first time—which he had to borrow—loaded the pockets with stones and managed to meet the minimum requirement.

He was trained as a commando and sent on the most rigorous kind of maneuvers designed to toughen him up. For example, he

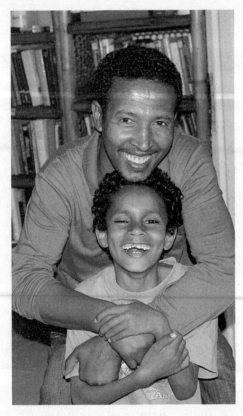
Bayelign, the former child soldier, with Danny in Rick's house.

said, they would be given one bottle of water that was to last for twenty-four hours and told there would often be no water where they would be fighting so they had to get accustomed to rationing their supplies. He remembers being hungry all the time. He was trained to shoot a gun and was given a knife to use when he ran out of bullets. "I was a good soldier," he says. "I wasn't afraid. I killed many people."

As a scout he conducted night commando raids in Eritrea for two years. At one point, he and his buddy Abraham were caught behind enemy lines at night and were sure they'd be killed. They devised a plan: they stole some cattle with big horns, tied hay around the horns, and set it on fire. The animals ran back to the villages. The enemy, thinking Ethiopian commandos were about to burn down their villages, followed the flames while Bayelign and Abraham made their escape.

But when the Ethiopian army lost the war with Eritrea, Bayelign jumped on an Ethiopian naval vessel that sailed into the Red Sea. The Yemenis refused them landing rights and he ended up on a desert island under the jurisdiction of Saudi

Arabia, where he lived for two years with three thousand other refugees from the war. Despite all of that, Bayelign says he would fight again to win back Eritrea, the land where he says his ancestors are buried, the land he believes is rightfully part of Ethiopia. He said his forebears, barefoot and using nothing but primitive spears, managed to keep the country together. Now that the Ethiopians are armed with modern military equipment, he thinks they should be able to reunite the country.

There are numerous studies and programs designed to rehabilitate child soldiers and bring them back into their communities. Disarmament, Demobilization and Reintegration, DDR, as it is called, provides psychosocial support to psychologically deprogram child soldiers who were trained to be killers. But Bayelign was reprogrammed in a novel way, the Rick Hodes way.

When Bayelign told Rick he couldn't read or write, the kids in the house taught him the alphabet and he started school in third grade. "Imagine, sitting at the age of twenty with third graders?" Rick said. "I don't think I could, but Baye did it." Bayelign was able to help Endale with Bewoket each time Rick had to leave Addis.

ALTHOUGH RICK HAD BEEN SKEPTICAL about how beneficial surgery might be for Bewoket, he finally found doctors in Atlanta willing to operate on him. In 1997, Bewoket's heart valve was repaired, but he wasn't out of the woods yet when Rick was pulled away from home once again. Two more JDC missions were being set up, first in Albania and then in Turkey.

One program was established for refugees from Kosovo in Albania, partly out of gratitude for the large number of Jews saved by the Albanians during World War II. The refugees from Kosovo were living in miserable conditions in Elbasan, about ninety miles outside of the capital of Tirana, sleeping on the floors in shelters with leaky roofs. "We quickly found people to repair the rooftops and found a factory that agreed to stay open twenty-four hours a day to produce ten thousand mattresses, which our team bought and distributed," Rick said.

Rick directed a number of clinics that had been struggling and also ran a training program. "I called my teacher from Johns Hopkins and told him I was finally practicing East Baltimore primary medicine," he said. "Everyone was fat, hypertensive, and diabetic. We hired local doctors, and I got an Albanian medical license."

He gave lectures and distributed medical books, especially the *Merck Manual,* one for each clinic. Then, once the immediate emergency was under control, the team tried to enrich the lives they had saved.

"As Jews we value education, so we started libraries," Rick said. "Other NGOs would call and ask for books and then ask 'how much?' They were amazed when they learned it was free."

Rick commuted between Ethiopia and Albania for about six months, sometimes staying for three weeks at a time.

"While I was there a well-dressed, middle-aged woman knocked on the door of our JDC compound and said, 'I want to see the Israeli doctor.'"

Rick told her he wasn't from Israel but asked if he could help.

"I just wanted to see the Israelis," she said. "My father saved forty Jews during World War II."

Rick asked the woman if his service had been acknowledged. She got in her car, went home, and returned with a plaque and a medal from the Israeli government.

A rare example, perhaps, of international cooperation on the human level. Beyond that, Rick said the work of the JDC as well as support from the government of Israel "demonstrated to the Albanian government the value of the Jewish community, which was able to mobilize aid from around the world."

6

I'LL TAKE THE KIDS

THE JDC SOON HAD RICK ON the road once again. His next assignment took him to eastern Turkey in 1999 when a huge earthquake caused devastating damage in Anatolia. Israel sent in a crack team trained to find victims in building collapses. "As for me," Rick said, "I'd like to say I helped bring people out alive, but the fact was I brought out the dead." He said he would remember for the rest of his life that, even with the most effective respirators, the stench was unbearable. "I had to stop every three feet and move away to get a place to breathe, even while all the time telling myself this is someone's child, this is a soul."

Upon returning to Ethiopia, Rick fell into a daily routine that was, for him, somewhat normal. He continued to shuttle between Addis and Gondar, where he called at the clinics set up by the JDC, which, now that Operation Solomon was over, were still treating the remaining Jews who were hoping to emigrate, as well as Ethiopians of all religions.

From time to time he was pressed into making house calls. One day he was asked to look in on Solomon, a young man who had worked at the JDC clinic in Addis for five years, who was gravely ill. He had been given a series of drugs for Kaposi's sarcoma, but he was not improving.

Rick says that in the Talmud it is written: "It is the duty of every man to visit a person who has fallen sick," and he wanted to see this young man, whom he'd known as a colleague. He says in the Jewish tradition, "Each visitor is said to take one-sixtieth of the illness away from the ailing person" (Leviticus). Proper attention to the sick is so important in the Jewish religion that there is an entire body of Hebrew texts devoted to the subject. There are, for example, specific directives in the religion for visiting the sick, including how to pray with them, whether one should sit or stand, what days are best to call on them, and even on how to speak to the sick and on what subjects. The Talmud says "one who visits the sick is saved from the judgment of hell."

Rick had no idea where the ailing man lived and with whom, but a nurse told him he was renting a room in a compound owned by his grandfather, a very nice room with a wooden floor and electricity and a solid roof. Relatives had come from the countryside to care for him. Rick set out with his nurse, and they found Solomon in a room about twenty by twenty-five feet, with dirty blue walls and a sign, written on tape, that read "God Is Love." Tacked to the wall above the bed was a poster of a kitten with a key in its mouth. It was captioned: "When God closes one door, he opens another."

The patient's brother walked over to the bed and nudged

him. "Solomon, Solomon, wake up. Your doctor is here."

Solomon took several minutes before he was able to turn from his stomach to his back and uncover himself enough so that Rick could see him. "When he did," Rick said, "I was shocked by the difference two months made in his appearance. He had lost weight, his eyes were sunken back, and his Kaposi's spots were still clearly visible."

Solomon was too weak to sit up, so he lay back on a pillow.

"I sat facing him with my foot on a nearby cabinet," Rick said. "He reached over and held on to my calf. I rested my hand on his leg. Physical contact is soothing, even healing. We chatted about my recent trip to Israel and the weather in Ethiopia, about how the clinic was not doing well without him and about local politics. After ten minutes, we saw a visible change in his mood, he became more animated and smiled a bit, his energy level picked up, and his eyes looked less glazed."

Rick's mind went back to the Talmud, which teaches,

The essential feature in the religious duty of visiting the sick is to pay attention to the needs of the invalid, to see what is necessary to be done for his benefit, and to give him the pleasure of one's company. Also, to consider his condition and to pray for mercy on his behalf.

"I did not think there was much I could do medically for Solomon," Rick said, "but I thought I should examine him, if only to invoke the magic of 'laying on of hands.'"

Rick then switched to his nonmedical mode. "How about school?" he asked. Solomon had always been a good student. "I've been writing away to schools," he said, pointing to catalogs

117

from British universities. "I hope I can get a scholarship. When I get better, I want to continue my studies. Both accounting and the Bible."

"Great," Rick replied.

He stayed another forty minutes, then got up to leave. He shook hands with Solomon's mother and brother, and then sat down on the bed for a moment and placed his hand on Solomon's chest. Rick recalled the statement of the Hebrew sages: "If one visits the sick, but fails to pray for mercy, he does not fulfill his religious duty.

"'Solomon,' I said, looking into his eyes, 'may God bless you and heal you.'

"'Thank you, Dr. Rick,' he replied.

"As I walked out, I looked up at the poster. 'When God closes one door, he opens another.'

"Solomon looked at me and asked, 'Doctor, the poster, it's true, isn't it?'

"'True,' I replied, 'one hundred percent.' I winked at him as I walked out."

After the visit, Rick acknowledged how impotent he feels in such situations: "I would like to do something grand and save his life or extend it significantly. Instead I ended up playing with ear drops and thinking about what we had spoken about and what we had not spoken about.

"Should I have brought up deeper topics? What does the Talmud say? 'They who visit the sick . . . should speak in such a manner so as neither to encourage him with false hopes, nor to depress him by words of despair.'"

Solomon's brother followed Rick outside. Rick was sure he knew his brother was dying of AIDS, but in Ethiopia many things remain unsaid. In America, technical issues of AZT doses and ventilators and schedules take on great importance. In Ethiopia, such issues are simply not pertinent. Instead people stay together, visiting, supporting, awaiting the inevitable end. Quietly.

"I was happy I had come to Solomon's home," he remembered. "It clearly had boosted his spirits, and that is perhaps the most important thing I could have done. As a doctor who feels much more comfortable defeating death (yes, sometimes we are successful) than making life's demise more calm and pleasant, I welcome situations like this with a bit of trepidation as a way of opening myself up to life's uncertainties, to develop an attitude of kindness and compassion.

"In the end I always feel I should do more, even though I realize there is nothing more to do. When death comes, I always feel an aching and hollow calm and a bit more appreciative of life, at least for a moment."

BEWOKET'S CONDITION WAS still troubling Rick. Ultimately, he had to send the boy back to Atlanta for lifesaving surgery to replace his damaged heart valve in 2001.

But before that, Rick felt the boy should see his family again, despite his continuing anger and sense of abandonment by his mother and father.

Rick sent his Ethiopian assistant, Berhanu, to Bewoket's village to search for the family, expecting that the boy would be recognized by the photograph he was given to carry with him. Bewoket's father couldn't believe his son was not only still alive but somewhat better. His older brother Chani was suspicious that this was some kind of trick cooked up in the big city. But he finally agreed to travel to Addis with Berhanu, where the brothers had a tearful reunion after a five-year separation. Soon the parents came as well.

"I told his father and mother to visit whenever they wished, and that I would pay for their trip," Rick said. "In this way they could actually make money."

So in the course of one of his visits, Bewoket's father told Rick about another of his sons who so desperately wanted an education that each night he lit a tiny oil-flame lamp and read in the semidarkness. "He wasn't asking for help," Rick said. "But I thought, here's a kid who deserves a chance."

There was an obstacle. Addisu was what in Ethiopia is called a cowboy; that is, he was caretaker of the animals, the family's main source of wealth. If he left the countryside, there would be no one to do the work. "I told them if they would hire somebody else to do the job, I would pay him," said Rick. To this day, this still costs Rick $1.00 a month.

At about the time Rick was thinking of taking in Addisu, one of the boys in the house had gone off to a boarding school in the southern part of Ethiopia. Rick called a family meeting because he could not stand having half a mattress free on the living room floor. He had space for another kid, and it was going to waste. The boys went through a list of candidates. One was rejected, then another, and another until finally Rick said, "What about Bewoket's brother, Addisu?" He said that because none of the boys knew him, they could find nothing objectionable about him and the decision was made.

"So Addisu comes to live at our house," Rick remembers. "He'd never seen a lightbulb or an automobile. He had never seen a white person. This was September 9, 2001. I enrolled him in first grade. Then he did second, fourth, sixth, and eighth."

One evening after dinner, Rick started to ask Addisu what it was like to be a kid growing up in his village. "Rick," Addisu interrupted him. "Stop right there. There is no such thing as 'kid.' I mean, the idea of childhood does not exist. You're a baby, then you take care of the animals. That's very important; it supports your whole family."

Any mention of Addisu prompts a couple of Rick's favorite stories. "Whenever I go to the States, I go to Costco and buy a hundred pairs of white socks," he said. "Every kid gets a few pair. I wear them all the time, even when I'm in a suit. Sort of a family uniform. Now, enter Addisu: 'Rick, you always buy white socks,' Addisu told me. 'You should buy black socks. They don't show the dirt, and you can wear them for three days if they don't smell too bad.'"

Then there was the time Rick said to Addisu, "You know, Addisu, Jesus was a Jew."

"Jesus was a Jew?" Addisu said. "Jesus was a Jew? I thought he was Protestant!"

Addisu's passport says he's eighteen now, and he looks like an Abercrombie model, a tall, strikingly handsome, ponytailed, soccer-playing, English-speaking eighteen-year-old studying at the Olney Friends School in Barnesville, Ohio, and hoping to qualify for a soccer scholarship when he goes to college. Because he is one of the only kids in the house without any health issues, Rick likes to say he snuck in.

—ᴍ—

ON ONE OF THE DAYS when he was walking through the dormitories at Mother Teresa's, Rick saw two little boys with severely deformed spines sitting together on a single cot. Dejene, the younger of the two, was an orphan who never knew his father, whose mother and then grandmother died when he was very young. The sisters in charge of this particular dormitory told Rick that an uncle had abandoned him, a five-year-old with a crippled back, at the door of an Orthodox Christian church.

Now a strong teenager with piercing eyes, Dejene speaks very softly in passable English. He still remembers how his uncles were walking along the road, carrying him and talking among themselves about where they would set him down. "I wanted to cry out, 'Don't leave me,' and when they placed me at the entrance to the church, I was stunned and just sat there for ten minutes, unable to utter a sound. Then finally I started screaming." After a priest found him and cared for him, he was fortunate to end up at Mother Teresa's mission for the destitute in Addis.

Not long after Dejene got there, another tiny, crippled boy was placed in his dormitory. That was Semegnew, a very small twelve-year-old who was so traumatized that he could never talk about what had happened to him or how he came to be there.

Rick says he can only speculate about his background. "He suffered a lot," said Rick. "He never mentions his previous family; he had no hope for the future and he was in pain all the time. I do know that he got on a truck and told the driver he had no money but he had to take him to Addis Ababa. Upon arriving in the capital, he started wandering around the city. He once said,

'I just followed my feet wherever they led me.' His feet eventually took him to Black Lion, the university hospital, where he slept on a slatted bench for sixty days while he was given daily injections for TB of the spine. After two months they sent him to the mission where I found him."

Semegnew was so frightened that he refused all food and just sat there and cried all day. Dejene took it upon himself to watch over the older boy. Semegnew would eat only when Dejene brought him food. Soon they started sleeping in the same bed to comfort each other. When Rick came upon the two of them—with their matching crooked backs—sitting on their cot, he started treating them.

Eventually he took them home. Now there were four living with Rick (in addition to Bayelign and Endale, who helped when Rick was away): Bewoket, Addisu, Dejene, and Semegnew. But the two younger boys needed surgery, without which their tubercular backs would collapse, severely compromising the spinal cord and the lungs. Their breathing would become more labored and they would die an agonizing death. But Rick had no means to get them corrective surgery, so he started a painstaking and sometimes discouraging search for a hospital that would treat them and perform the necessary surgery.

Rick sent medical studies of the two boys to doctors around the United States until he finally found a hospital that would agree to operate on them as demonstration cases. But he would still have to pay thousands of dollars for any medical expenses that might occur outside the hospital. That's when he came up with the idea of adopting the boys so they would be covered by the medical insurance he receives as an employee of the American Jewish Joint Distribution Committee.

But it meant that the "price" for getting the boys lifesaving surgery was for Rick to be their father for life. "I was not thrilled with that much permanence in my life," Rick said, but then he reminded himself of the religious texts. *God,* he thought to himself, *is offering you a chance to help these boys. Don't say no.*

Adoption was not an easy process. The Ethiopian government did not permit single males to adopt, but Rick went to the authorities about the boys, who were already living with him and Bewoket and Addisu anyway. So he made his case to the government, fortunate that he'd come to know many of the officials in the course of his work with the Ministry of Health and the orphans' bureau.

"They came to interview us," Rick recalled. "We had dinner in our house, and the guy saw I was a normal guy and the kids were normal. Then he took the kids aside for a few minutes and talked to them." Rick says the officials concluded that he was an okay guy, a man to be trusted.

"In December 2001," Rick said, almost as if it was an everyday occurrence, "I adopted them. Sem was fourteen and Dejene was seven or eight."

But it was a momentous decision, particularly for a loner like Rick, who was now taking on the permanent and inescapable responsibilities of a single parent, a turning point in his life. Even Rick probably did not grasp the full implications at the time. The official adoption of two boys, even more than taking in Bewoket, set the course for the rest of his life. He was now a father; he took to referring to his boys as "my babies." And the boys affectionately refer to their Jewish grandmother, Rick's mother, as *bubbe.*

Rick's own grandmother, Rose, remained unmoved. "My

grandson is a jerk," she told her doctor. "He should be making tons of money like all you guys. Instead he's living in Ethiopia."

Rick's newly adopted sons, Semegnew and Dejene, were accepted for surgery at the Scottish Rite Hospital in Dallas, but that presented yet another problem. Rick couldn't move to Texas for a month and neglect his work in Ethiopia to be with them. So, as he remembers it, "I called the *Dallas Jewish Week* newspaper to take out an advertisement to explain my situation and ask if anyone would help.

"I told the story to the advertising department, and the woman said, 'Doctor, this is a wonderful story, but you're wasting your money. Don't bother taking out an ad. Call Jewish Family Service. There's a woman who knows everyone and everything; call her and ask her for her advice.'

"I called the woman, Jaynie Schultz, and left a message. An hour later when she called back I told her the story and asked if she knew anyone who might be interested in helping with the kids. She immediately said, 'Oh, I'll take the kids.' They lived with her for six months."

Another reason Rick believes in miracles.

BY THE TIME THE BOYS RETURNED TO ADDIS, Rick was setting up something that began to look like a real household with regular family rhythms. Now there were his two new back patients in addition to Bewoket and Addisu, as well as Bayelign, Endale, and Dereje, a student who had started living there. So there were seven in residence, but even that didn't last long.

Soon Rick brought Mesfin Yoseph to the house. "Mesfin came to Mother Teresa's on his own, to die," said Rick. "He felt he was causing his family too much suffering. He was so weak he couldn't walk across the room and gasped for breath."

Mesfin's story is typical of those of many of Rick's kids, so it's worth looking at the autobiographical essay he wrote for his high school American literature class by way of thanking his benefactor for the happy ending to the twists and turns of his life:

> *It seems I have already lived my entire life. . . . I was born happy like anybody else, with a large family, the fourth of thirteen brothers and sisters. I was born in southern Ethiopia in a small village without electricity or automobiles but we never lacked for love or family closeness. We were happy with what we had. I could have lived my entire life in that naturally beautiful village, but I became dreadfully sick and my life took a different course. An unexpected complication from a sore throat caused an infection to my heart, and it began to fail.*

Mesfin said that when he was younger he had been able to walk four hours a day to and from school, but then he became so weak he couldn't walk across the room. "I could never get to sleep; every day I coughed and was short of breath. It became increasingly difficult to perform simple daily tasks."

Three years of tribal medicine did him no good. "By then I was at the point of death, and I was praying to be delivered from my suffering. I was not afraid to die, for I had lost my hope to live. Struggling to breathe, it felt like I was drowning all the time. I gave up hope, but my parents never did. They were sure I would live, and yet they didn't know how. I guess that is what you call faith. It's their greatest gift to me."

By the time Mesfin was fourteen, he felt he was becoming too great a burden to his family. "They stayed up every night with me as I struggled to breathe," he wrote. "When I hurt, they hurt. I felt my family was dying with me."

The young boy decided he should die alone and made the long journey to Addis Ababa. "I left the village to go to Mother Teresa's Mission, a place for people to die.

"While I was at the mission I met this man whom I called 'my angel.' His name is Rick Hodes."

Rick knew that if Mesfin were to survive, he would need heart surgery, and he started contacting hospitals across the United States for help. Mesfin was finally accepted in Atlanta, where a philanthropic group, the Children's Cross Connection Organization (CCCO), found a host family and paid for his trip and his surgery.

"In order to prevent serious heart infection, they pulled out my wisdom teeth," Mesfin wrote. "They gave them to me. In my culture it is the custom that when your teeth are removed they should be cast in the exact place of your birth. But I decided I loved America and its people so much that I would give my teeth to my second birthplace, America."

Mesfin returned to Ethiopia, but his ordeal was not over yet. "Very unexpectedly my mouth became infected," he wrote.

The infection spread to my heart, and before I knew it, I was dying again. My "angel" Rick came to my rescue again and arranged the flight back to America. The am-

*bulance took me to the emergency room, but I can't re-
member it at all. They repeated the heart surgery by re-
placing my heart valve and after that I was given a new
American family. My American dad just happened to be
my cardiologist! My new mom is a nurse, and I have four
new brothers and four new sisters.*

*See, I already have lived my entire life. However,
in the middle of trouble lies a good opportunity. I was
blessed with a second life to live, to grow, to go to school,
to be happy with my American family and great Samari-
tan people. I love my family and friends as well as the
country. Again and again, I say, "God Bless America!"*

With Mesfin in America, another vacancy opened at Rick's.
It was becoming dangerous for Rick to go to Mother Teresa's; he
kept returning with new boys.

Before long Rick brought home another Mesfin (a popular
name in Ethiopia), an abandoned child who had been placed in
a room for sick, unadoptable kids at Mother Teresa's. When he
was a very small boy, he was out walking with his mother and
watched in terror as a car ran into her. With his mother dead,
his stepfather took him to Addis and set him down on a sidewalk near some boys who were playing marbles. Just left him
and walked away. He was one of the lucky street kids; he ended
up at Mother Teresa's and then Rick took him in.

But soon the boy ran away, obviously frightened that he
would be abandoned once again. They searched for him for
two nights and finally gave up. "He knows where we are," Rick
told the other kids. "If he wants to come back, he will." He
did. Rick started sending out e-mails looking for someone to

adopt him, but when no one came forward, Rick adopted him instead.

Now there were eight mattresses strewn on the floors each evening—for Bewoket, Addisu, Semegnew, Dejene, Dereje, Bayelign, Endale, and Mesfin.

But Rick wasn't finished yet. One day he was walking through Mother Teresa's when he saw Mohammed, a young boy who had lost his right leg to cancer. He was hanging out with Temesgen, another child about the same size who'd also lost a leg, the left. Here were two more matching boys, like Dejene and Semegnew. The two had become inseparable, and both needed chemotherapy, so Rick took them home and administered their intravenous medications on the front porch on Sunday mornings.

Now there were ten.

When he took the two new boys to buy shoes, he found they could share a single pair because they were the same size. "I took this as a message from the Almighty that they are a couple," Rick quipped.

One day while they were both having chemotherapy, Rick overheard Temesgen ask Mohammed what he told his school friends who asked how he'd lost his leg.

"I tell them I had cancer," he replied.

Temesgen said, "You told them you have cancer? I'd never say that. I tell them I was in a helicopter accident!" Rick savors the incongruity of the story.

When Temesgen first came to him, Rick wrote down his diagnosis: "Temesgen is a 10-year-old boy with osteogenesis imperfecta who was breaking his bones every three weeks."

Rick consulted with a doctor at Johns Hopkins, who advised him to administer pamidronate.

"It costs $3,500 a year," he said. "I did not have the money."

One day when Rick was leading rounds at Mother Teresa's with a group of medical students, he showed them Temesgen and said, "Now I have to find pamidronate. It's made by Novartis."

The moment he said the word *Novartis,* someone tapped him on the shoulder. "It was a tall white guy I'd never seen. I asked if I could help him. 'I was walking by and heard you say Novartis,' he said. 'I work for Novartis.' We exchanged information, he contacted the right division, and sent me a two-year supply of meds."

This went down in Rick's mental notebook as another miracle.

Temesgen got the medicine, stopped breaking his bones, and started walking for the first time in years. The medication extended his life and gave him time to have further treatment in America. He was taken in by a family in Washington, D.C., where he was provided with the best available medical treatment for metastatic osteosarcoma. But sadly, all efforts—including experimental protocols—failed, and he died in September 2008.

Mesfin Hodes told a grieving Rick, "Dad, God wanted him but too early." Rick recalled another loss, Abraham, whom he took home from Mother Teresa's when they were unable to provide chemotherapy there. Rick treated him in his living room for lymphoma, but he couldn't save him.

"I think Abraham was an angel who came down to earth and has now returned to where he belongs," Rick says wistfully. "Anyway, I gave him a shot at life, and nobody else had attempted to do that. It's the best I can do. When they die after some meds and a good fight, then I somehow feel that it's an act of God. If they die without any effort (which is often, because nobody will bother doing anything for them), then it becomes a tragedy and life becomes worthless."

By this time, Rick decided to offer a place to Teshale Yoseph, the younger brother of Mesfin, who was remaining in Atlanta. The plan was for Teshale, who has no medical problems, to go to a private school in Addis and then join his brother in Georgia. But in a heartbreaking twist of fate involving the breakup of an American family, it didn't work out that way, and Teshale will probably have to stay in Ethiopia. He is living at Rick's and going to school, but his ambition is to make movies, not the kind of work that's easy to find in Ethiopia. He's an ardent admirer of Angelina Jolie—teenage boys are the same all over the world—who became especially popular in Ethiopia after she adopted a child there. Denzel Washington is another of his favorites.

The count was now nine, and Rick started looking for a bigger house. The walls wouldn't stretch any farther. He found a ranch-style house with three bedrooms and a four-room servants' quarters in the back. Of course that only meant he had space for more.

Just then, Zewdie showed up at the clinic where Rick was examining patients. The boy had started feeling pain in his back when he was four years old. It got progressively worse, and his spine started becoming deformed. His family was wealthy, as they tell it; the father's family had a big farm with five oxen, four cows, seven or eight sheep, and two donkeys. His mother says she was "*very* rich"—four oxen, four cows, horses, a donkey, and ten sheep. They took Zewdie to a traditional healer, a person of some fame in their region, who lived three hours away. Zewdie's father worked for him for three days, and in return the boy was given one traditional massage. Not surprisingly, it did not help at all. Nor did a local hospital, which apparently started him on treatment for tuberculosis but did not provide the full course of medication.

When that hospital could do no more, Zewdie's father sold two of his sheep for 300 birr and took the boy to Addis Ababa by bus, the fare about a quarter of what he earned from selling the animals. They found a hotel where they were allowed to sleep on the floor, without blankets, and were directed to Mother Teresa's, where Zewdie was examined by Rick.

Rick remembered that the first time he met them he gave the boy tablets for eight days and ordered x-rays. "I gave him one red pill to take each day. And 100 birr for rent."

"Were you surprised?" Rick asked Zewdie's father.

"*Betam, enji,*" very surprised. "Nobody can lend us that much money, much less give it to us. Nobody."

"I saw that these were very poor people," said Rick. "Zewdie, with an angle over 120 degrees in his low back, a collapsed chest and a huge draining lymph node in his groin. . . . In this condition they were walking six miles each way to get to us to save the bus fare, and they were eating one *injera* a day to save money. I told them, 'I will give you 100 birr every time you come here. So use this money. Spend it. Eat. It's okay.'"

Eventually, Zewdie moved into Mother Teresa's and then into Rick's house. He reported to the mission each day for his medications. "The key to TB control is compliance," Rick said. "This is accomplished by DOT: directly observed therapy. Each dose is supervised." Once Zewdie was cured of the disease, Rick knew he would have to find someone to perform surgery on the boy's back. Meanwhile, Rick told Zewdie's father to visit any time, and every few months he would show up.

Rick never knew whom he would find sleeping on the living room floor when he awoke in the morning. At this point in his life, people came and went. Some stayed; some were cured and moved on. Some died. He grieved and he prayed, but as long as he was making the effort to help, he was a happy man.

7

MY SON HAS BEEN REBORN

Not long after Zewdie arrived in 2005, a local teacher in Addis asked Rick to look in on a patient who had developed an infection following back surgery. Rick contacted the surgeon, a Dr. Oheneba Boachie-Adjei in New York, and they exchanged e-mails about the case. In one of his e-mails, Rick said he was coming to New York to see his father, and Dr. Boachie suggested they meet. So it was that because a boy in Addis happened to develop a postsurgical infection, Rick came upon an extraordinary doctor who was ready and able to help his growing number of patients with spinal deformities, Zewdie among them.

Connections within the philanthropic medical establishment tend to be serendipitous and unpredictable. Groups and individuals who may be willing to help are hidden in pockets around the world, but most of them know little or nothing about the others. Finding Dr. Boachie meant Rick would no longer have to scrounge around and send out multiple letters hither and yon looking for help, at least for his spine patients.

Dr. Boachie invited Rick to his office at the Hospital for Special Surgery, one of the best orthopedic hospitals in the United States.

As Rick remembers it, the walls of his office were filled with awards and framed articles about his work, but he felt the many accolades were not necessary to know that this man, who headed the spine service at one of the world's most prestigious orthopedic hospitals, was a substantial physician. There was something in his manner, Rick says. "He is soft-spoken and low-key. He does not brag. He does not have to. You know he is probably the best spine surgeon in the world."

Dr. Boachie was born in Ghana, and when he was eight years old, a Western-trained physician cured him of a tropical disease that otherwise would have killed him. He vowed to help others, and to repay the favor, he returns to Ghana twice a year to perform surgery on needy African children at no charge. He operates in a government hospital, although he has been working for years to raise funds to build a state-of-the-art thirty-bed facility there. A dignified compact man with a neat beard and aristocratic bearing, he has started a foundation, FOCOS, the Foundation of Orthopedics and Complex Spines, to help children with spinal malformations.

The two doctors ordered in pizza, and Rick told Dr. Boachie about his work in Ethiopia and described the kind of help he needed. Rick explained that he had no money, but Dr. Boachie

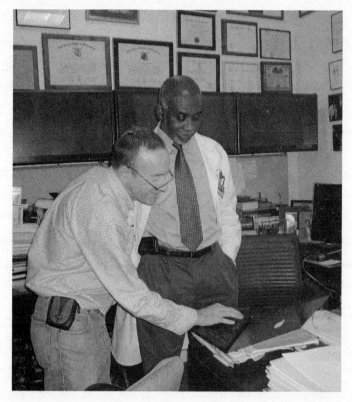

Dr. Oheneba Boachie-Adjei with Rick in his office at the Hospital for Special Surgery. They are selecting from the long list of candidates waiting for back surgery.

didn't consider that an insurmountable obstacle. He said, "Let me know about your funds, and we can figure out how to work together."

Rick now had a link to a lifeline for his kids. If he could raise enough money for air tickets plus hospital costs—$10,000 for each child—Dr. Boachie would take up to twenty of his patients every year. This meant even that the poorest of the poor would get the finest medical treatment in the world, operations that could cost $100,000 and more in the United States.

Dr. Boachie followed a unique path to hone his craft. When he decided he wanted to be a spine surgeon, he took a year off to work in a pathology lab where he dissected two hundred spines. "Nobody had ever done that," Rick said. "He wrote a book about the pathology he saw, taught himself to remove vertebrae, and worked on cases that nobody else could handle."

He does not aim for perfection, which in back surgery is truly the enemy of the good. "I don't go for a home run," he says. "The downside is too great. A double or a triple is fine. This is not cosmetic surgery." But it is a balancing act. Too much correction and there is a danger of paralysis, even death. The surgeons go for 50 percent, to straighten the back without damaging the spinal cord and to allow the lungs to expand properly to permit normal breathing.

Whenever Dr. Boachie goes to Ghana, he brings a large team of volunteer surgeons and nurses who pay their own way and work without compensation to learn from this great man. Doctors from some of the finest hospitals in America and around the world work twelve- to fifteen-hour days in crowded operating rooms under miserable conditions. The electricity goes out at least once a day and often stays out for hours. That means that in the ninety-plus-degree temperatures of Ghana's capital, Accra, the doctors work without air-conditioning and often without lights. Dr. Ken Paonessa, from central Connecticut, who has volunteered to go several times, says he once had to finish the last forty-five minutes of an operation using only miner's lights, which sent a beam onto the patient from the lamps on the doctors' helmets.

Although the conditions are better in Ghana than in Addis, even necessary equipment is often unavailable.

"Rick," Dr. Boachie said when they first met, "our kids get malaria from transfusions. Can you find us a donor to buy a cell-saver?"

"How much money are we talking about?" Rick asked.

"Thirty-five thousand dollars should do it," he replied.

"I'll check eBay," Rick said dryly, "and I'll ask around." Or, as he would have told his kids, KD, Keep Dreaming!

When the volunteer doctors finally finish their work for the day—which is often after 10:00 P.M.—they return through bottlenecks of traffic that choke the Ghanaian capital at all hours to a FOCOS guesthouse where they sleep on double-decker beds and contend with unpredictable showers and iffy meals.

Yet even with all of this, they are positively ebullient after their long day. With each patient presenting unique complications, the surgeons develop inventive ways to cope. The doctors bring new procedures with them and often end up taking others home.

"There is a huge value in having the infrastructure and two or three surgeons looking at one patient and collaborating to solve problems together," said Dr. Michael Mendelow, a surgeon from Detroit. "Here one and one make three. I've seen that so many times working in Ghana. What we're able to do together seems to have a multiplier effect."

On that first visit, Rick brought along studies of some of his patients, and Dr. Boachie selected five of them for surgery. As Rick's luck would have it, a philanthropist from Dallas was about to visit him in Addis and would provide funds to jump-start the process. This turned out to be a spectacular Christmas for Rick; a true gift had been given him, the chance to help more patients.

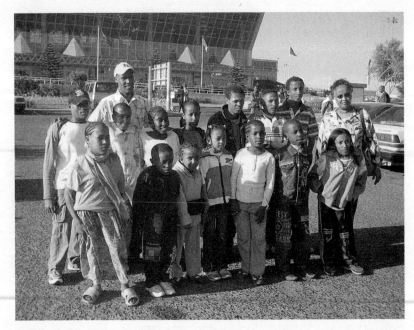

Here are some of Rick's patients at the airport getting ready to leave for surgery in Ghana. They are accompanied by Berhanu and Sister Tena.

Zewdie was one of those accepted for surgery in Ghana and went off with Rick's first group in 2006. All did not go well. The hospital had a severe water shortage, and the Boachie team had to cancel six surgeries. Zewdie was one of them.

"Zewdie was bummed," Rick said. "He sat. He cried. He wondered if his back would get worse or he'd become paralyzed. Dr. Boachie sat with him and said, 'Listen, Zewdie, there has to be a reason why this happens. Let's make the best of this. You are here. This is your chance to help the other kids.' Zewdie took that message to heart and ran with it. He was at their bedside all the time. He fed them. He called for help when they were in pain. He held their arms as they were walked. Dr. Boachie promised him: 'Next time, you're first.' He was."

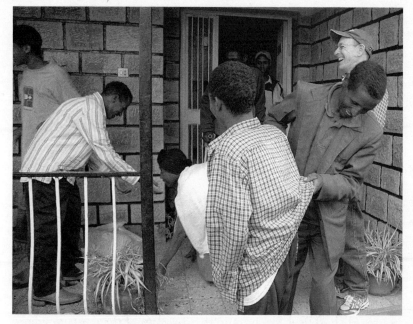

"My son has been reborn," Zewdie's mother screamed the first time she saw him after his back surgery.

After Zewdie was home at Rick's for a few months, his parents came to visit him. Zewdie's mother arrived wearing an immaculate greenish blue cotton dress that went below her knees. No shoes. She had short-cropped hair and was wearing a large cross. It was her first time in Addis Ababa. She had never seen a white person before. She had never seen TV.

"I asked one of the kids to run in the back and get Zewdie," remembers Rick. "When Zewdie stepped out front and his mom saw him, she let out four or five short, high-pitched screams: 'whew, whew, whew, whew.' She held her hands up in the air and she turned around several times and she shouted, 'Look, look, my son has been reborn.' She kissed him several times. Then she kissed his feet, a sign of respect. Then she turned and kissed my feet in excitement. Teshale was standing next to me. She kissed his feet. He ran away, not wanting his feet to be kissed."

"At one point," Rick recalls, "I explained to Zewdie's dad that Dr. Boachie's team operates without charge, but it is still necessary to pay the hospital costs and the local doctors in Ghana. Zewdie's surgery cost $10,000, or about 90,000 birr, for airfare and food and accommodation. 'Do you have 90,000 birr to pay for this,' I asked half jokingly. His dad smiled. 'Listen,' he replied, 'I don't have 90 birr.'"

"I take it as a personal challenge," Rick said, "to send patients all over the world for care, at no cost to them. I have to raise about $10,000 for each spine patient in Ghana, which is about 5 percent of the cost of the same surgery in America."

By this time, a boy named Tesfaye had also moved into Rick's house. He had been sleeping in the shadows of the *merkato* where he was a street vendor, what Ethiopians call a *souk b'deretee*, "a store around the neck." He wore whatever knickknacks he had to sell on a string. The boy's back was one of the most deformed Rick had ever seen; he likened it to a dinosaur's. Dr. Boachie had him brought to Ghana so he could examine him himself but determined that he could not do the surgery there because the kind of anesthetic it would require was not available there. Rick eventually found a doctor in Vancouver and a donor who was willing to pay his fee of $60,000 and to provide him a home while he recuperated.

Rick has an ever-growing list of patients who need surgery and is always looking for more sources of medical support like that provided by Dr. Boachie. If he could raise the money, in addition to the two groups he sends to Ghana for spine surgery, he'd send two groups a year to India for spine surgery and two

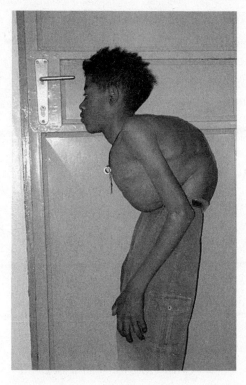

Here is Tesfaye, who had one of the most deformed backs Rick had ever seen.

groups a year to America and India for heart surgery.

"You get into visa problems and, of course, money," Rick says. A half a million dollars a year would cover this wish list, but he is now able to raise only about $150,000 a year for these projects. The JDC allocates $800,000 each year for Ethiopia, a sum that includes Rick's salary. Beyond that, says Rick, "We've gotten people to sponsor surgeries." One eighty-year-old woman in Kansas City who heard her rabbi speak at Temple B'nai Jehudah after he'd seen Rick's work in Addis said she wanted to contribute $7,000 as a birthday present to herself. That paid for a young girl's back surgery. The temple's youth group sponsored another back patient. Then the Methodist minister in the same city said his church also wanted to sponsor a patient. Employees of a law firm in Toronto sponsored another, and the Entoto Foundation in San Diego paid for two more.

Rick's work got a temporary boost when Morton Meyerson of the Morton H. Meyerson Family Foundation of Dallas agreed to match some contributions earmarked for Rick's patients who do not fall under the JDC rubric. "Only when people see where the money is going and that the money is well spent are they ready," Rick said.

On Christmas Day in 2008, help came out of the blue. A radiologist and his wife, who is a nurse, wrote a letter from Nebraska to say they were adopting four Ethiopian children the next spring and meanwhile wanted to send Rick $10,000 to spend as he saw fit, either on his patients or on his extended family. Rick was dumbfounded.

RICK ALWAYS HAS AN EYE OPEN for any chance to get help or raise money, even in the most unlikely places. Consider the elevator in the Sheraton Hotel in Addis.

The Sheraton on Taitu Street is the ne plus ultra of Addis Ababa, a grand luxury spa and watering hole for businesspeople and for diplomats who come to the headquarters of the OAU, the Organization of African Unity. (Around Addis it is known as the Organization of Useless Africans.) Outside the hotel, tin-roofed shacks are clustered along the streets, goats forage for the few blades of grass that grow on the side of the road, donkeys are laden with firewood, and sputtering taxis spew black exhaust. Inside the gate, the grounds are carefully tended and richly green; the swimming pool beckons, fountains are programmed to "dance" to piped-in music. Every now and then, one of Rick's pals who lives there will be traveling for a day or two and offer the room to him for a vacation from his own cramped quarters. On one of these occasions, when the Boeing representative and his wife had gone off to Rome and the room and breakfast for two would have gone unused, Rick was invited to stay there. Whenever this kind of bonanza falls into his lap, he takes a different kid with him as a special treat—real beds with crisp sheets, a marble shower, croissants! One night, when he was returning from work at 11:00 P.M., he encountered a white woman in the elevator and, just to make conversation, asked what she was doing in Addis. When she replied that she was part of a medical team doing facial and heart surgery, he jumped at the chance to inquire whether they had enough patients. "Too many heart patients and not enough facial patients," she replied.

Rick had just the person for them. "At that point," he said, "I had a woman with a huge facial tumor who had been waiting for surgery for years." So he met the team for breakfast at the hotel and asked them to come to the clinic the next day to examine some of his patients. They immediately agreed to operate on three of his cleft palate patients as well as the woman with the tumor. There were only two complications. First, they needed a neurosurgeon to participate in the surgery and, second, they needed a CAT scan. Rick quickly found a neurosurgeon, John Clark, who was visiting from Utah. He agreed to work with the surgical team. The CAT scan wasn't so easy. It was a weekend, and one could not get a CAT scan until Monday. Monday was Yom Kippur, the Day of Atonement and the holiest day of the year for Jews, a holiday strictly observed by the Orthodox.

So here was Rick's dilemma: "I asked myself, should I go to synagogue (and possibly be the tenth person for the minyan for my community), or work with this woman? You can guess—I spent the day (wearing sneakers—you don't wear shoes on Yom Kippur) praying and transporting my patient around. By the end of the day, we had new x-rays and a CAT scan, and two days later, she had successful surgery."

Rick is that rare on-the-ground link between the millions spent on medical care in the developing world and the delivery of that care to the patient, the nexus that is often missing. Jim Yong Kim, then a professor at Harvard Medical School (and currently president of Dartmouth College), who with Paul Farmer founded Partners in Health, told Harvard medical alumni at a symposium in 2007 that "each year at least ten million preventable deaths occur around the world. . . . The most critical roadblock in delivering care in the developing world is not money, but an implementation bottleneck." Thousands more Ricks would be required to clear that bottleneck, and except by example, Rick is pretty much a force unto himself. He encourages medical students to come and work with him, and they do, but only for a summer or a single term, and then they go home. Rick is a unique phenomenon that cannot be replicated or institutionalized. There are other lone wolves around who are also doing good works, but far too few to meet the need.

Rick is nevertheless trying to expand his reach. A windfall $1.1 million grant from the Osher Foundation in Texas is being used to build schools, dig wells, send children abroad for heart surgery, and allow three doctors from Baylor Medical School in Texas, one a year, to work in Gondar under Rick's tutelage, starting in 2009. "This is how I started in Ethiopia," Rick says, "but when I went on my Fulbright there was no one there to guide me. Now I will be their mentor. It will be like passing the baton." He says the three visiting doctors will increase the pediatric capacity in Gondar by 200 percent.

Every year, Rick has also worked with volunteers and has

become a mentor to many of them. Zvi Kresch, now in medical school, believes he speaks for dozens of others when he says that after a year in Ethiopia, he is excited about the idea of continuing with international medicine. "I will say that as I get more toward clinical practice, I'm pretty much using skills I developed in Ethiopia and attribute to a mentor like Rick."

In the best of all worlds, Rick would try to do even more. He is always saying if he wins the lottery or the Power Ball he would like to establish a hospital for poor children in Addis where he could care for them and train doctors and health workers in what is known in the trade as a "resource-poor environment." He also is brainstorming a scheme to encourage American children to raise funds. "If I could get two hundred children to each raise five thousand dollars through charitable projects or by contributing money from their bar mitzvah presents," he says, "I could have a million dollars to provide medical care to needy Ethiopians."

Meanwhile, he spends each day treating whoever comes his way, one by one, no matter how hopeless. He is ever mindful of what he learned in the refugee camps. "I must not make choices. I must treat whomever God puts in my path."

In the Talmud, Rick likes to say, Rabbi Yeshua Ben Levy asked Elijah the prophet where he could find the Messiah. "He's at the gates of the city, dressing the wounds of the lepers, one by one," the holy man replied. Rick reflects that with everything else the Messiah has to do, aside from rebuilding the Temple, aside from returning the Jewish people to the ways of Judaism, aside from bringing peace to the world, he was spending his time treating the lepers. "So maybe what we're doing is pretty important after all," he says.

This is not to suggest that Rick has a Messiah complex, but he revels in this story and it makes him happy. He would not have the temerity to compare himself to the Messiah, but he knows that what he's doing is—in his typical understated manner—somewhat important. He is saving lives, many of them, and he is also living by the precepts of the Bible and the Talmud, which fills him with satisfaction and pleasure. He's no Messiah, but Boaz Bismuth, that Israeli reporter who gave blood to a dying woman during Operation Solomon, says that in his entire career, he never met an angel like Rick.

8

IF I HAD A HAMMER

Rick's now quite large family in Addis was developing its own rhythms and traditions, chief among them the weekly celebration of Shabbat. As an observant Jew, Rick celebrates all the holidays, even the most obscure ones, but he particularly rejoices in the Sabbath.

His Friday-night gatherings have become *the* place to be in Addis for any visiting foreigners, assorted denizens of the diplomatic community, and, of course, Rick's kids. This is the one evening when the entire family gets together. But what goes on at Rick's house is not exactly the ritual one might expect from a devout Orthodox Jew.

"Shabbat shalom," Rick says, looking a bit like a skinny leprechaun in a skullcap. "This is our house," he tells the Friday-night

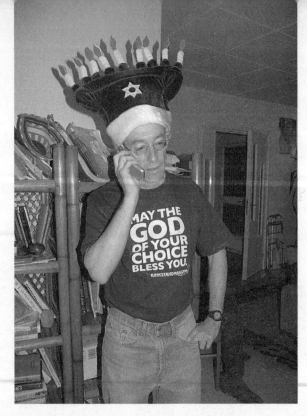

Rick at his Shabbat service during Hanukah, 2007. He wears his sincere piety lightly.

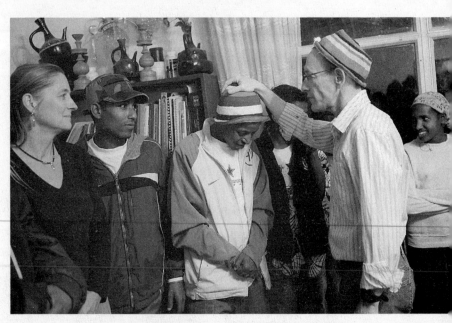

May god give you peace. Rick blesses all the children at the end of his Shabbat service, lingering a bit longer with his adopted children.

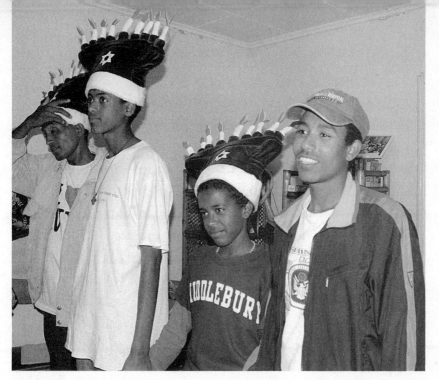

At the opening of the Shabbat service, Rick asks everyone to join hands and sing "If I Had a Hammer"—all of the verses.

Dejene, Mesfin, and Rick decked out for a Shabbat service during Hanukah, 2007.

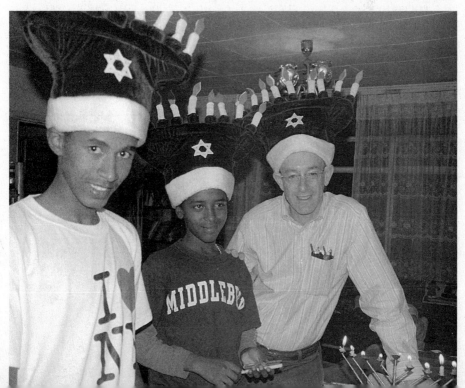

guests who squeeze into the shabby living room. "It's crowded, and it's not very clean, but we like it that way."

When foreign visitors come, they get a taste of the unusual within an exotic country. And these evenings provide an opportunity for Rick's kids to spend time with people from faraway places who have different talents and professions. It's a chance for them to see a world beyond their own experience.

Unlike many Orthodox Jews, Rick wears his piety lightly. He has a T-shirt with the saying MAY THE GOD OF YOUR CHOICE BLESS YOU, and occasionally he puts it on for the Shabbat service, a far cry from the black hat and *payess* associated with his spiritual brethren. He asks everyone to join hands in a circle to sing Pete Seeger's "If I Had a Hammer." The song has been adopted at some Passover Seders because it suggests freedom from slavery, and for Rick it brings a bit of Americana abroad and, he thinks, creates a nice feeling of goodwill.

The older boys reach into a sack and distribute their growing collection of funky hats, and Rick, in a wonderful tenor voice, offers the traditional prayers in English and Hebrew and invites everybody to sing Sabbath songs. He breaks off chunks of the Sabbath bread and tosses them to one and all. At the end of the ceremony, he walks around the circle to each of his kids, lingering just a bit longer with the sons he has adopted. As he puts his hands on each of their heads, he prays in Hebrew: "May God bless you and keep you and give you peace."

Then everybody crowds into the small kitchen where huge pots of soup and stew, known as *wat,* and a buffet of pasta, beans, and vegetables, are set out to be wrapped in the inevitable *ingera,* the grayish spongy pitalike bread that is fairly unappetizing to foreigners but much loved by all Ethiopians. It all disappears quickly. There is a continuous din of chatter and laughter until the kids bed down for the night on sofas, on mattresses dragged in from the porch, or, for a lucky few, in real beds.

The kids' main wish, as they drift off, is that one of their many foreign visitors will find a wife for Rick—a tall order considering that any woman would have to take on the entire package, including all the kids and, regrettably, Rick's room, where decades-old reports and x-rays are piled to the ceiling, and his bathroom, where he stores another set of archives in the bathtub. He seems totally oblivious to what can charitably be called a unique filing system. He claims to have "a general sense of the archaeology."

What woman would take on all of that?

And still, Rick was accumulating more kids.

Tihune came in 2006. She had been brought to Addis from Gondar by a woman, who had promised to get her treatment for a severe spinal problem but instead provided no medical care and put her to work in her house and the houses of her friends. Tihune said she felt she was being made into a slave so she ran away and went to Black Lion Hospital to see if they could cure her twisted back. They said they couldn't treat her, but suggested that she go to Mother Teresa's, where she would find a doctor named Rick who deals with bad backs.

Rick had just made the connection to Dr. Boachie and was able to send Tihune with the first group that went to Ghana for surgery. But during the operation, she suffered neurological damage and needed constant care, so when she returned to Addis, he felt obliged to take her into his house.

"She couldn't use her left leg for some time and she needed to be in a sheltered place," Rick says. "So she became the first girl

I took in. She could barely walk from the front door to the gate." It took about a year before she was back to normal.

Rick wasn't at all sure about bringing teenage girls into the house to live side by side with teenage boys. But there has never been a hint of a problem. "We see ourselves as brothers and sisters," Addisu says.

Asmara Lewtu was twelve years old when Rick found her in 2006. She was abandoned in the hospital at Gondar and had been living there on her own, without family, for an astounding three years.

As Rick remembers it: "I was walking along the grounds of the hospital, and because my interest in spines is known, she was pointed out to me."

He saw that she was at a good age to intervene, and he arranged for her to come with him to Addis and live at Mother Teresa's. She stayed there for quite some time before being sent to Ghana for surgery. As he got to know her, Rick realized she could hardly see, so he gave her a pair of his own eyeglasses, with his minus 8 prescription. This helped some, but she was minus 12 and needed something stronger. Eventually he got the proper correction for her, and her world changed overnight.

When Asmara returned from having surgery in Ghana, the nuns decided there was no longer any reason for her to live at the mission, and Rick, seeing she was bright and could do better in life than her probable future as a housemaid, found a place for her in the house. Now there were twelve children at Rick's. Asmara wants to be a doctor, a high-value profession in the Hodes household.

Zemenewerk, a twelve-year-old who is the size of a six-year-old, is the child Rick literally bumped into as he was walking to an Internet café to check his e-mail, when he was unexpectedly delayed in departing from Gondar, a city of 130,000 that is just a step up from a village. Rick still can't get over the uncanny workings of fate. He recalled, "As I was headed to the Golden Internet Café, I took two steps, and right in front of me, I saw a young man with a small girl who had a twisted spine. We almost collided. I took one look and saw that she had a bad back. I notice this in a split second these days. TB spines are part of my daily life. My home has at least eight kids with serious spine disease, some operated, some not."

He stopped the young man accompanying the little girl and said, in Amharic, "She has a bad back, no?"

"Yes," the man replied. "Terrible. And the doctors here say it is hopeless. Her back gets worse every year."

The young man, who introduced himself as Menormelkam, the girl's uncle, spoke in broken English and told Rick they'd gone to the hospital where each doctor they saw had a different theory about how to cure her. "One doctor said that perhaps they could squeeze her in a certain way and her back would become straight. Another said they could give her a pill and this would straighten the spine. A third said there was an easy operation to help."

Then, after being told to wait five days for a diagnosis, another doctor looked at her x-ray and said there was nothing that could be done, that it was far too late.

The man said they had spent the family's last birr and were just now looking for a place to sleep before taking their disappointment back to Belesa, a remote village in the countryside that had four huts with mud walls and grass roofs. He and the girl had broken down in tears when they were told there was no hope, and they were still crying when Rick ran into them.

Rick, in his somewhat limited Amharic, told the uncle, "I treat people like this," he said. "I send them abroad for surgery."

Rick took the little girl into the corner of the Internet café to examine her back, but when he pulled up her dress, he saw that she was not wearing any underwear.

He said, "I wanted to give her some privacy, and didn't want to undress her in front of strangers, so I took them back to my hotel room. I saw that she was very small, extremely thin and her back was twisting, more prominently on the left. I wanted to listen to her chest. She was afraid. I asked the uncle to lift his shirt so I could listen to his heart, and she could see that it is painless. That worked.

"'Listen,' I said, 'I can't promise anything, except that I'll try to get her help. She needs tests that can only be done in Addis Ababa. I'll find a place for her to live.'"

With that, Rick handed the uncle 300 birr, about $33—a fortune for a man who had exhausted the family's savings to bring the girl to the hospital.

"Of the eighty-two million people in Ethiopia, I believe I'm the only person who could possibly help Zemenewerk," Rick said with not a small amount of wonder. "I should not have been in Gondar anyway on Wednesday; I was there only because I extended my trip. There was only a fifteen-second window for us to meet—the twenty-step walk between Delicious Pastery [*sic*] and Golden Internet."

"Rick, this is a miracle," said Teshale, who had come to Gondar with him and saw the story unfold.

"Watching the news that night, I saw that our encounter took place on the tenth anniversary of Mother Teresa's death," Rick said. "I bet she's looking down at us, smiling."

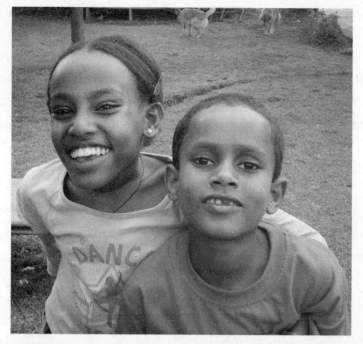

Zemenewerk and Danny. Zemenewerk has never lived like this. She has earrings. She goes to private school and studies hard.

Zemenewerk's mother died when she was three years old, and her father abandoned her to her grandparents, who used her as a servant. Only the uncle, her mother's brother, made any effort to help her. From the moment she came to Addis, she began living at Rick's. Until there were enough beds, she slept on the right end of the couch—with Tihune at the opposite end. She had new (or perhaps gently used) clothes. She had earrings. She was slowly getting used to her new family.

She is also going to private school like all the other kids, and Rick keeps a running check on her to determine the cause of her illness.

"I am very concerned about her lack of growth," Rick

said. "I'm giving her nutritional assistance and will start zinc chews."

A year later, Rick at last got a diagnosis. Zemenewerk suffers from spondyloepiphyseal dysplasia, a form of dwarfism, and Rick has begun seeking ways to treat it—if there are any. In the meantime, Zemenewerk's life is on the upswing.

"She never lived like this," says Rick. "It's very amazing. She says she loves it, playing with the kids, the food, a bed."

She's always smiling and she studies hard. She has become one of the house favorites, almost a sort of mascot, and she performs a mean professional-quality shoulder-shaking traditional Ethiopian dance.

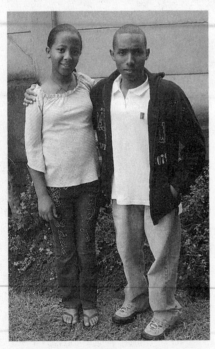

Balemlai with her brother Zewdie, who was doing so well at Rick's that his father asked for his sister to be allowed to come and study.

Zemenewerk is very close to Balemlai, Zewdie's sister. When Zewdie's father saw how well his son was doing, he asked Rick to allow his little sister to come to be educated. Rick was delighted that in this male-dominated society, a family wanted to give a daughter the same opportunity it was giving a son.

So many kids lived at the house now that people began to mistake the Hodes compound for an orphanage. The front yard always seemed filled with girls wearing blouses with longish skirts, the boys dressed like teenage boys everywhere, jeans and oversized T-shirts imprinted with the usual, but in this environment bizarre, advertising logos, most of the clothes hand-me-downs brought to Addis by visitors who collect huge mounds of clothing from neighbors before they come.

One day when I was visiting, Mesfin was wearing an unusual T-shirt. On the front I could see the face of a small child peeking through a large *V.* I asked him who it was, and he hadn't a clue. I asked him to open his buttoned shirt and there I saw, printed on the front of the tee, the words I PLAYED THE WIENIAWSKI CON-CERTO WHEN I WAS FIVE.

I asked him to turn around so I could see the rest of this intriguing shirt. On the back was written 60, and I suddenly realized that this shirt had been handed out to guests at Itzhak Perlman's sixtieth birthday party and that I had sent it to Addis for the kids. (I didn't think I'd be wearing it a lot around Manhattan.)

The shirt gave me the opportunity to tell Mesfin about Itzhak Perlman, the story of how as a child he was crippled by polio but had never ever been handicapped by it, and the way, to this day, he walks on the stage, sits down, unlocks his leg braces, and plays like an angel. I told them that he'd become one of the great violinists of the world.

Mohammed was listening and became become quite emotional about the Itzhak Perlman story. He was almost in tears as he thanked me for telling it. This is the young man who lost his right leg to cancer and uses two canes. He, like Perlman, recognizes no handicap.

"Did you play soccer today?" Rick asks him.

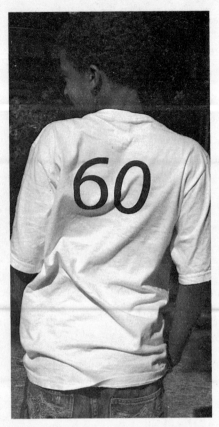

Mesfin wearing Itzhak Perlman's birth-day shirt.

"Yes," he said.

"With one leg?"

"No, with three," he said, holding up his two walking sticks as he balanced himself perfectly on his left foot. His upper body muscles—his arms, his back, his chest—have become incredibly powerful from using those canes, so much so that he looks like he spends hours lifting weights at the gym. He says he wants to become a doctor so he can find out what causes cancer.

Looking at him as he propels himself forward at impressive speed, Rick comments, "Mohammed is as bothered by having one leg as I am by a hangnail."

RICK LOVES KIBITZING WITH THE KIDS, but even for him the day is only twenty-four hours long, and the work tends to crowd out both the joys and the duties of parenting. There are unspoken rules that are strictly enforced in his house: no lying, no cheating, no stealing. But he readily acknowledges that he has no idea how often the kids change their (white) socks or take showers, and he manages somehow to blot out the noise and disorganization that surrounds him. He provides the shelter, the food, and the tuition, and he seems to figure the kids can take care of one another and that the house will run on autopilot.

"We don't get to see enough of him because he travels so much and is always working," says Addisu. "He works the whole day at the clinic and works at home and leaves before we get up in the morning. He's always going to the mission or going to see somebody who's sick. Sometimes you don't see him for two days."

That's hardly surprising if you consider just one of his to-do lists, the kind he makes up every morning:

- Check with New York for possible surgery.
- Write to a potential donor about her idea of importing sandals for peasants to wear to prevent podoconiosis (silica-induced elephantiasis).
- Meet a patient with TB spondylitis at the post office at 3:00 P.M. to give him 350 birr to return home to Tigrai, now that we've finished his tests.
- Fill in the financial aid form online for two of my kids who want to go to boarding school in Ohio.
- Write to a Congregational minister in Boston to thank her for her donation and for informing me that I am John Irving's Owen Meany without the voice.
- Do CMEs at NEJM.org.
- Research how to treat a new patient with non-Hodgkin's lymphoma.
- Ask an endocrinologist about interpreting the increased gonadotropin levels and low testosterone in a twenty-five-year-old with micropenis and possible Klinefelter's.
- Write to the U.S. embassy to get a medical visa for a

four-year-old patient with an abdominal mass who has the opportunity to go to America for treatment. She has a psoas abscess after full treatment of TB.

- Look for second-line TB drugs on a four-year-old Ethiopian girl who may need retreatment.
- Choose a growth hormone preparation for my son Mesfin, based on stability if refrigeration goes off.
- Look for the really smart orphan at Mother Teresa's Mission who speaks English and Hindi and just arrived from N. Shewa, and sign him up at a private school for next year. Find a donor for $1500/year for this purpose.
- Order books online for an Ethiopian doctor friend.
- Send a centrifuge from Addis Ababa to Gondar and order a new one for Addis Ababa.
- Give pamidronate to my patient with osteogenesis imperfecta this week, go back to the older dose (1 mg/kg for 3 days) due to bone pain.
- Finish tests on my ten patients with spine disease and send by UPS to the surgeon in New York. Review the manuscript for my friend's book.

Occasionally Rick adds to his own workload by making forays into the countryside to look for sick people. He frequently goes to Lalibela, the ancient city with the fantastic stone churches carved into the rock, where 80 percent of the inhabitants are infected with trachoma. What is extraordinary about this disease, however, is that it can be cured with a single dose of azithromycin. Whenever he goes there, he fills his pockets with tablets and walks through the town where he might stop an old man limping along with the help of a thick pole, lift an eyelid, and, where needed, dispense the medicine along with a swig of water from a plastic bottle. Then he stops another and another, lifts an eyelid, offers the medicine. With this fifty-cent pill, Rick is able to prevent blindness.

Jake Tabel, an American medical student who has gone to Addis several times to do volunteer work with Rick, once said, "I think he would object if I were to describe his purpose in Addis Ababa as humanitarian. His work both begins and ends in Africa—this is his home—and so he differs from most people involved in humanitarian work, who have the security of knowing there is a more comfortable place to which they can always return."

Rick once tried to describe his unique existence in Addis in a letter to a friend:

> *Let me give you a glimpse of my life. It is 2:00 a.m. I took a nap around midnight and now am trying to get a bit of work done. It's raining like hell. In the poor neighborhoods everyone is awake because of the noise of the rain pounding on their tin roofs. . . . My house has rats. My toilet does not flush. My computer crashed today; I went back to my old computer. The floor of my bedroom is filled with piles of medical journals, x-rays, MRIs, and papers.*

Nevertheless, Rick says, with not a little sense of wonder, he is happy—or at the very least content and fulfilled. Despite countless frustrations and frequent disappointments—and the heartbreak of seeing some kids die—he revels in his everyday life.

With his phone always ringing and the chaos of kids everywhere, Rick has no privacy in his own house, but he allows himself one luxury—membership at the Sheraton Hotel fitness club, where he swims a mile a day every day. It keeps him trim and clears his head. Then he comes home, the aroma of chlorine and soap still trailing him (a good thing, since his bathtub is brimming with those piles of records), sleeps very little, taking only a catnap when his eyelids start to close, and spends most of the night on a hard chair in the corner of the living room roaming the Internet—when he can get a (slow) connection—e-mailing those digitized x-rays and medical reports and looking for doctors around the world willing to consult. (And he says he never lets a visiting student leave without a body part—a biopsy, a slide, an x-ray, or a CAT scan—to hand-carry to a doctor in America for evaluation.)

Through the Internet he keeps himself au courant on all the news in America and around the world and monitors his own Google link to "Rick Hodes," which indexes any and all references to himself. As a man who works unheralded in the obscurity of Ethiopia, he is not offended when he finds his work has been noticed.

Would this suggest that the good doctor has a streak of self-importance, after all? An egotist, perhaps? Maybe, but if so, this is one of the only signs of it. Just as likely, he is searching the Internet for fund-raising opportunities. Any money contributed to the JDC specifically for Rick's work goes directly to him without administrative costs. The more money that comes in, the more he can help his patients.

And the more doctors he can recruit. He is always on the lookout for more people like Dr. Boachie who will accept some of his patients. Whenever he goes to the United States, he makes it a point to meet doctors who have responded to his requests for advice, and he is always happy to be invited to do rounds in their hospitals. In this way he forges relationships with the medical community in the service of the many patients who make their way to his door.

In 2008, he spoke at MD Anderson Hospital in Houston, Texas, because of an e-mail relationship he's had for years with a physician there who has given him unpaid advice on patients. During grand rounds, some of America's best cancer specialists literally gasped when Rick presented slides of some of his cases. One doctor asked how he manages to finance his work. His answer was simple, if only partly true: "I beg," he said.

9

EVERYBODY GOES TO RICK'S PLACE

Rick holds clinic every Friday and Saturday in one of two small spartan rooms outside the chapel of Mother Teresa's mission. Nestled behind a blue-painted metal door on Sidist Kilo, the mission is a small enclave of low stucco bungalows painted turquoise or apricot or blue or tan with corrugated tin roofs that shelter hundreds of men and women behind gracefully arched windows. Across the street there is another series of dormitories for mothers and children as well as a separate orphanage. The six hundred or so sick or dying indigents pass their days mostly sitting on the bare ground, their legs stretched in front of them. Those who can, shuffle about the walkways in various stages of lethargy, many of them on crutches. Most of the men are unshaven, dressed in faded pajamas and worn-out slippers and wrapped in grimy shawls; the women, too, wear shawls, these draped over cotton housedresses that look like they are cut from one very large bolt of cloth. There is a constant hum as they gather in the fetid compound for wound care or form a queue to see the only resident doctor. At mealtimes they line up for their food and sit on the floor in the hallways to eat out of tin plates. There is no cafeteria. To amuse themselves, kids throw crumbs in the air to attract birds, which obligingly swoop down to create an impromptu performance.

When Rick arrives on any Saturday, he drives through the blue gate and jumps out of his dusty station wagon, hat askew, stethoscope around his neck, his arms loaded with his laptop, a supply of pills, and a few x-rays. He long ago came to terms with the idea that Shabbat restrictions against working can be violated if necessary to save a life.

Patients are already waiting to see him, the American doctor who has become something of a legend in Addis. There are the children with life-threatening heart disease, teenagers with crazily crooked spines, young adults with faces hidden behind shawls to cover grotesque tumors that distort their faces—all of them on pilgrimage to their own personal Lourdes. One boy, ravaged by Ollier's disease, had hands grossly disfigured by huge tumors that made each one look like a medieval mace. When Rick took him to the U.S. embassy for a visa to go to America for surgery, the consular official took one look at him and could utter only two words: "Jesus Christ!"

There are more of these people every day, some of them even arriving by way of a unique referral system typical of the genuine care Ethiopians tend to show for one another. Recently, for example, a woman jumped off a bus when she saw a boy with a deformed spine. "Go see Dr. Rick," she told him. In some ways, this city of four million is like a village.

In 2006, the JDC added Rick's volunteer work at Mother Teresa's to its official program, allocating an additional $150,000 a year to its nonsectarian activities in Ethiopia, which also include building rural schools and providing clean water.

There could be no greater example of the overwhelming need than a heartbreaking scene I witnessed one afternoon at Mother Teresa's. I was standing in the garden when I saw the blue gate pushed open, the gate that separates the home for the destitute from the utter misery that is outside. A small child, maybe a year old, was prodded inside and the gate pulled closed behind him. He stood there, alone, looking around, not knowing which way to turn. The guard came over and gently guided him back outside. Seconds later, the gate was cracked open again and the little fellow was nudged inside again. Finally, the sisters were called. They found the child's young mother huddled outside and referred her to an orphanage. She was trying to do something both simple and shattering: find a safe place to abandon her child. It happens every day.

Ethiopia has recently become a favored destination for Americans who want to adopt children. The hotels are full of couples with small Ethiopian boys and girls dressed up in the clothing that the proud new parents have brought for them, the children sitting in the dining room on the many high chairs that have been readied for them, eating strange new foods with small delicate fingers. Perhaps, in part, it is the influence of Angelina Jolie and Brad Pitt, who adopted an Ethiopian child; perhaps it's just the availability of so many children in need. The World Health Organization estimates that there are four million orphans and abandoned children, many of them left alone because their parents died from AIDS; UNICEF puts the figure at five million and, in addition, reports that 13 percent of children throughout Ethiopia are missing one or both parents. Now, with famine once more threatening throughout East Africa, it will only get worse.

ONE SATURDAY RICK WAS BEING assisted by Dr. Irving Fish, whom he'd found at the Addis airport when he was picking up patients returning from surgery in Gondar. When Rick learned that Dr. Fish was a pediatric neurologist, he dragooned him into coming to his clinic at Mother Teresa's to consult on some of his most difficult neurological cases. Today Rick is in the nine-by-thirteen room that is painted a sunny yellow and embellished with matching yellow cotton curtains. He is somehow comforted by the idea that this particular room is, at other times, used for confession.

A plaque on the door says, "I shall pass through this world but once. Any good thing that I can do or any kindness that I can show to any human being, let me do it now and not defer it, for I will not pass this way again."

Betelhem, who had surgery in Ghana for scoliosis, has returned for a checkup. Rick reflects that he can sometimes cure the disease, but he can't cure the poverty that brings it on. With this patient, he is concerned that she is getting proper nutrition, which is especially important after surgery. There's reason for him to be worried. Betelhem's mother tells him that when people give them money, they eat; otherwise, they don't. She explained that she had been laid off from her factory job where she was paid 15 cents for each kilo of plastic shoes she produced. Rick has been paying the girl's school tuition, and on this day gives the mother what he calls "bus money," which he knows will allow them to buy food for a week. "Come back next week," Rick tells them, "and I'll give you carfare again."

Dr. Fish, who has seen Rick reach into the pocket of his khakis to shell out money to almost every patient, tells Rick he ought to think about closing early before he goes broke.

"He's the only doctor I've ever known who pays his patients," Dr. Fish says.

Rick recalled that when Betelhem first came to him three years before, he had chatted with her mother while some American medical students looked on. "Here was a mother who made less than a dollar a day. I give her money for transport. I make sure that I don't have change, so she gets far more than the buses charge, making her life just a bit easier." At that time he asked about her son, a boy of five. When the mother explained that she had the opportunity to send him away for an education, Rick, always curious about ways to improve prospects for children, asked for more details. Then, as if a light went on, he suddenly realized she was giving the boy up for adoption in Italy.

"I felt terrible," he said. "Like the heart-wrenching scene in *Seabiscuit,* she could not afford to support him so she was giving him up. I asked if she had been paid. Not one centime. It really hurts me to see parents giving away their kids like this. I shook my head in silent pain."

At just that moment Rick's son Semegnew unexpectedly arrived at the clinic while Rick was thinking out loud to the students. "I mentioned options: what if I paid the mom $20 per month?" he mused to them. "What if I agreed to enroll him in school as well? Why should I intervene? Should I play God? There are so many like this . . .

"'Sem,' he continued, 'is in boarding school in America, with his eye on the same college I attended. By nature he's quite shy.' But he looked up and interrupted me. 'Rick,' he said firmly, 'you're wrong.' I turned and faced him. All the students looked at him.

"'What are you thinking?' I asked.

"'Look at the circumstances,' he said. 'Look at what's going on. What will happen if he stays here? Give him a chance in life. Come on.' I paused to consider the situation, astounded by the synchronicity of events. Sem never shows up at the mission on Saturday mornings. Now he walks in just as I was to make a major decision about intervening in the life of my patient's mom.

"I paused for a moment, then looked up and said, 'Thanks, Sem. Let's see the next patient.' Saturday clinic continued."

But it didn't end there. The impoverished mother began to have second thoughts. When final legal steps were under way and the boy was about to be given up for adoption, a judge asked her if she understood that he was going away and she might never see him again. She had convinced herself that he was going away only for an education and would return. When she realized what she was about to do, she reneged. Now Rick not only sends Betelhem, his former patient, to school. He sends her brother as well. And the mother is regularly given "carfare."

—᚜᚛—

FETIA SHOWED UP AT THE CLINIC with hydrocephalus and a cleft palate just a week before a team of facial surgeons was arriving from Detroit in early January 2008. Her mother had taken the six-year-old girl with a severely distorted face from one hospital to another and could not find help anywhere. Then she was told about Rick and searched for him for four days. Her timing was excellent, and Rick was able to send her to Gondar where the surgeons were operating. When she returned to Addis, Rick asked Dr. Fish to examine her to determine whether a shunt would help lessen the swelling in her head and relieve pressure in her brain. They decided against it (shunts can cause infection), but the mother was thrilled with the results of the surgery even though the child's face was still badly deformed. As they were leaving the clinic Rick called after them.

"Do you go to the mosque? Pray for your doctors," he said.

"I go to the mosque every week and pray for you," she replied.

The next week we went to their house, a hovel really, in traffic an hour's drive from the clinic, where we were welcomed with a traditional coffee ceremony. We watched as Fetia's beautiful mother lit the brazier and roasted the coffee beans to a perfect turn, and Rick joined in, asking to crank the grinder.

"Are you happy?" Rick asked.

"Yes, yes, are you kidding?" she replied.

When she left the clinic, Rick had handed her the usual "carfare," a gesture carefully noted by their sharp-eyed neighbor who had accompanied them. A month later the neighbor sent me an e-mail with a none-too-subtle request for money, and the next December she turned up at the clinic again, this time with a young student in nursing school who sought out Rick for financial help to finish his studies. Clearly, word was out that there was a guy with deep pockets over at Mother Teresa's, and she had brought this young man to get his hands (and maybe hers) on some of the money being handed out. I was incensed, but Rick was unperturbed. "I have no problem saying no," he says.

But he says yes very often, doling out carfare or juice or tuition or even a small business loan. He's running a mini-microfinance operation straight out of his pocket.

Sinteyehu Abayneh is five, looks like a three-year-old, and has a severely distorted tubercular back. His shorts are pulled up high on his tiny chest. He looks up at Rick with big round eyes as the doctor examines him with his stethoscope. Rick then goes into one of his favorite riffs.

"How many belly buttons do you have today?" he asks the child.

"*And*" (one), the boy answers.

"Oh, that's right, Ethiopians have only one," Rick says.

"*Farenge sa*—how about foreigners?" he asks. Rick runs his hand slowly across his own lower abdomen and answers, "Yesterday I had three; today I have four and a half."

After several days, most of the children claim to have several. Rick is hoping to get surgery for Sinteyehu's back. He's on his ever-growing list of candidates.

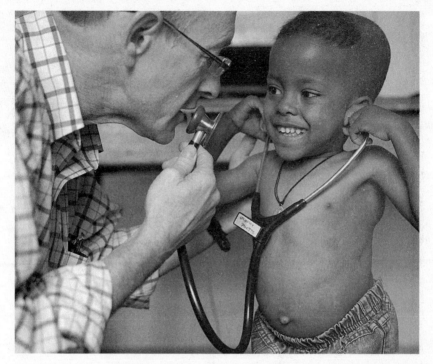

Sinteyehu Abayneh, a spine patient, in for a checkup and a little fun.

"There are a couple of things that can make these kids laugh," says Rick, who is always looking for new ways to put his patients at ease. "Ethiopians have only one given name; the concept of a family name does not exist here. To their names (which are frequently biblical names, like Daniel, or Amharic words that have a meaning, like Bewoket, 'by the will of God'), they add their father's given name, and their grandfather's given name, and so on, down the generations. (In the Ethiopian system, my name would be Richard Elliot Philip.) For example, I ask Bewoket his name, to which he answers 'Bewoket.' *'Bewoket man,'* 'Bewoket who?' I ask. 'Bewoket Sintayehu,' he responds, adding his father's name. *'Sintayehu man,'* 'Sintayehu who?' I ask. 'Sintayehu Abebe,' he

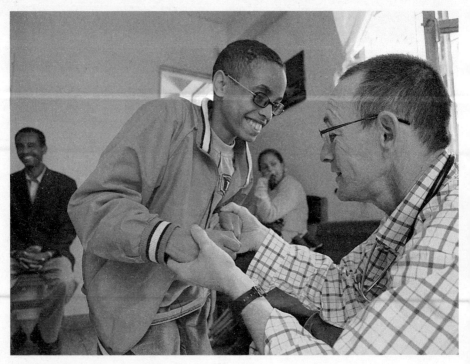

Do you dance? Matios being examined.

responds. At some point, often after six or seven generations of names, he will respond, *'Alawkum'* (I do not know). *'Alawkum man,'* I ask, as if *Alawkum* is simply another name."

So Rick has taken to referring to a patient as, let's say, "Mohammed *Alawkum,*" Mohammed I Don't Know.

"What's your name?" Rick asks the next boy, who is so crippled he has to be carried in by his father. "Matios," the boy replies. "Same as last week," Rick says. "You didn't change your name." The boy laughs while his mother sits in the corner, covering her eyes so we won't see the tears. "I really want to help this boy," Rick tells a group of students looking on. "Look how his parents love him. Both of them come every time, and the father gives up work to be here." To the translator he says, "Tell him he has a really good mother." Rick has asked Dr. Fish to consult on this case because not only does Matios have a severely deformed back, his legs are like Jell-O and won't obey his will to walk.

"Do you like television?" Rick asks the boy.

"Yes,"

"Music?"

"Yes."

"Do you dance?"

The boy laughs at the absurdity of the question while his mother weeps even more. Once the boy is at ease, Dr. Fish conducts a neurological examination and concludes that the boy most likely has cerebral palsy. He shows the parents how to help Matios do stretching exercises that will make him more limber and promises them that if they do it two or three times a day, the boy will feel better.

A few weeks later, Rick sends an e-mail to tell me he'd gotten some medication to improve the boy's mobility.

> *Great news. Remember Matios Dawit, the*
> *13-year-old with severe scoliosis and cerebral*
> *palsy who walks with crutches? His parents*
> *are so devoted to him, both show up at each*
> *appointment? I got hold of Baclofen and started*
> *it, and he tells us that he's significantly more*
> *flexible now. I'll follow Irving's advice on dosing,*
> *at present I just increased it from 10 bid to 10 tid.*
>
>   *He was just accepted for spine surgery in*
> *Ghana. One of the Ghana nurses was just here, and*
> *she wants him to stay a bit longer so that he can*

benefit from prolonged physical therapy after his
spine surgery.
We are really happy about this.

Matios needed a lot of extra help, so his father went with him to Ghana where he also lent a hand to the other patients. Matios can't walk yet, but a very happy-looking teenager in a wheelchair returned to Addis four inches taller than when he left. His back is straight, and he is continuing his physical therapy. Rick says he has given Matios permission to try walking. The latest news is that he can get around with a walker.

RICK PUT OUT A CALL for Atsede Gashaw to come over to the clinic from the mothers' and children's wing of the mission across the street. She is clearly a favorite of his and was being readied for heart surgery in America. Rick explains that she has severe heart valve disease, the result of a strep infection that led to rheumatic fever. She is such a pretty little girl that Rick has crowned her Miss Ethiopia. "This," he says, "is the next supermodel, right here."

Atsede arrives at the clinic accompanied by her mother, who is crippled by a tubercular hip and walks with a thick pole that serves as a cane. They clearly adore each other, and Atsede takes care of her mother rather than the other way around. "I want to send her to California if I can get her there," says Rick. As she leaves, she leans over and gives Rick a kiss on the cheek. He beams.

"Someone will find her a host family," he said. "She has been offered free surgery at Cedars-Sinai in L.A. and all she needs now is her air transport." It couldn't come too soon. In August, Rick got an emergency call from the sisters at Mother Teresa's that Atsede was very sick. "I dropped everything and drove to the mission," he reported. "She had been somewhat unresponsive, but neuro-intact. I suspected that she had gone into atrial fibrillation, but she was in sinus rhythm when I saw her. My son Addisu and I drove her all over, getting a chest x-ray, blood test, and EKG. One blood test was back at the end of the day showing a dangerously low level of potassium. I gave some oral potassium (I have it in the glove compartment of my car—there is none in the country right now), and she seemed okay. I left her an evening and morning dose, and I'll see her first thing in the A.M."

ONE SATURDAY A TALL MAN with an elegance undiminished by his grimy clothes led a small boy into the clinic. In fact, the boy with huge dark eyes and a mischievous smile was leading his father, who was blind. The boy, Lekune Negusse, had been brought to Addis as his father's seeing-eye son. Now the boy had come to Rick for treatment of severe scoliosis.

He wore a soiled black-and-white-striped T-shirt and a frayed knit cap that was unraveling. He never changes his clothes. He has no other. He never takes off his hat because it covers a huge scar from a burn that ravaged the left side of his head. And that's the least of his troubles. The father earns a living for the family— about 50 cents a day, but, he is quick to add, 60 or 70 cents on a holiday—while a brother, Mesfin, looks after their one-room hut (to call it housecleaning would mistakenly elevate both the work and the abode) before and after school.

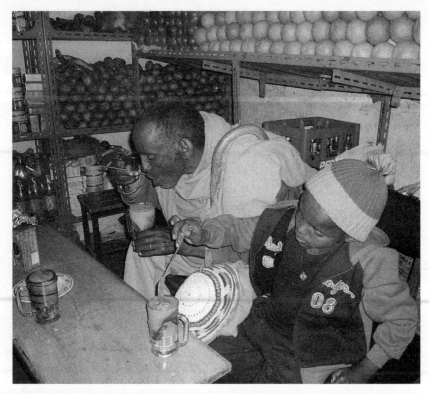

Lekune and his dad finally get something to eat. The boy saves a package of cookies for his brother.

Lekune, who is ten years old but looks considerably younger, oversees the care of his father, helping him to eat and to navigate the busy streets of Addis. Each day, before going off to school (where his father is proud to say his son is a very good student), he leads his dad to the corner that they have staked out, his place of business so to speak, where he stands all day with his hand outstretched. At night, Lekune retrieves him and helps him collapse to the floor onto their shared bed, after which he crawls in himself, wedged between his brother and his father on the foam twin-size mattress. Soon, the family of three will have to leave even this miserable bit of shelter. They are now paying their landlord $5.00 a month, but they have been told the rent is going up, so they will have to look for something more affordable, and probably even less adequate. Meanwhile, they sustain themselves with whatever food they can find, canvassing local restaurants for leftovers or begging scraps from neighbors and, as a last resort, checking the marketplaces for wilted produce the sellers have left behind as waste.

Rick invites Lekune and his father to the juice kiosk, and we watch as the boy ladles thick avocado puree into his father's mouth, like a mother with an ailing infant. When the boy is given a packet of cookies, he takes one and subtly slips the rest under his shirt to save for his brother. He leaves a third of his own juice in the glass and then gently feeds that to his father. Lekune says he wants to be a driver when he grows up. That way he would always have shelter and he would not be cold at night because he could sleep in the car. Rick arranged for the boy to have surgery in Addis for the burn on his head, and he is a candidate for back surgery next year. A benefactor has already volunteered to pay for it.

RICK WAS POSITIVELY DELIGHTED when he was able to arrange cardiac surgery for another patient, in California. For reasons that will become apparent, I will use a pseudonym for this boy, a five-year-old I'll call Eyob. The child was so cheerful and healthy-looking and busy with his Game Boy, you'd never guess he had a life-threatening heart problem. His uncle came to the clinic to report that they had been able to obtain a passport for the boy and that his mother wanted to go to the United States with her son. No one spoke about a father being involved with the family.

On the boy's next clinic visit, this time with his mother, they sat in the garden of Mother Teresa's. The mother dissolved in tears when Rick informed her she could not go with the child. This did nothing to soften Rick's resolve but instead made him angry and curt. Rick makes judgments, and his judgment in this case was that if the mother were to go to the United States, it would be very difficult to persuade her to come back, and Rick gives his word to the American embassy that his patients will not overstay their visas.

Within a week Rick had organized Eyob's departure, with his fare paid by the Entoto Foundation of California. He was to be accompanied by a college student on his way to the states. Rick arranged for Eyob's mother to say good-bye at the mission so there would be no tearful farewells at the airport, and Eyob stayed at Rick's for a few nights to become acclimated to being away from home and to become accustomed to the young man who would be his traveling companion.

Eyob underwent a cardiac procedure that is considered so uncomplicated that it is sometimes done at bedside, although in this case it was done in the catheterization lab. At first he was doing well, sitting up and eating Popsicles. Then he began to complain of abdominal pain, and a nurse noticed he had stopped moving his legs. An MRI showed a huge area of ischemic injury to the spinal cord, at approximately the midback. In non-medical terms, there was apparently a period of inadequate blood supply to a part of the cord and that caused his reflexes to shut down. The stroke team, the spine team, and others were brought in.

Rick was stupefied. "Paralysis after a simple heart procedure. Amazing," he said. "It's highly ironic that I deal with risk of paralysis from my spine patients, but now I'm dealing with paralysis in a cardiac patient?"

The only fortunate part of this story was that the nurse overseeing the child was Ethiopian, and she was able to call Eyob's mother every day with updates.

Now Rick had to arrange for her to fly immediately to the States so she could be with her son during his rehabilitation.

He was in the middle of dealing with a couple of kids with back problems at the clinic when he had to hunt down Eyob's mother so she could go to the airline office to pick up her ticket. When he finally found her, she was in church and said she couldn't leave. Rick handed the phone to his son Mesfin to be sure his message got through in a way the woman would clearly understand.

"Tell her that God is available twenty-four hours a day; KLM is only open this morning," he said.

This was the only moment of levity they could find in this situation.

The mother's flight to the states involved a seven-hour layover in Amsterdam and she spoke no language other than Amharic. Rick described to her the layout of the airport and handed her a note to give to any airport official if she had a problem:

PLEASE HELP ME TO TRANSFER FROM FLIGHT NW 8576 FROM ADDIS ABABA TO AMSTERDAM TO FLIGHT NW 8601 FROM AMSTERDAM TO LOS ANGELES, LEAVING AT 1320 PM ON 1 MARCH, 2009.

Eyob is said to be making some progress; he is showing signs of nerve regeneration. The hospital operated on Eyob gratis. It is now facing a malpractice suit.

YABTSEGA CAME INTO THE CLINIC for a postsurgical checkup and to show Rick his certificate in computer skills. He had come to Rick one Saturday when Berhanu was standing outside taking a break, something he hardly ever does. As Yabtsega walked by, Berhanu stopped him because his spine was seriously deformed. He immediately brought him into the mission so Rick could examine him.

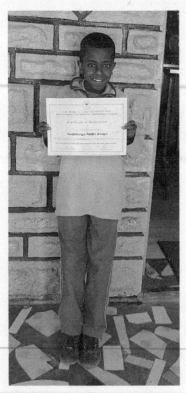

"I told the boy that he needed his mom's permission for me to take care of him," Rick said. "He checked and said it's fine. I treated him, gave him extra money so he could drink juice every day to fatten him up, and sent him to Ghana. He's fine now."

After Yabtsega recovered, Rick says, his mother was on a bus when out of the window she saw a boy with a terrible back, a perfect stranger, a Muslim boy. "She got off the bus at the next stop," Rick recalled, "and ran back to tell him he needs surgery and he should go to the mission."

After Rick arranged back surgery for Yabtsega, he sent him to school and the boy returned to show his certificate in computer skills.

The next Saturday, she went to find the boy and took him directly to Rick.

"You see how his hands go to the middle of his knees," Rick said, showing a digital photo of the boy. "He's squashed. This spine is unbelievable; they've never seen anything like it. If he doesn't have surgery, he will die through slow and terrible suffocation. This kid is a high priority for me."

One mitzvah leads to another. The boy, Mohammed Kemal, had surgery in Ghana in November 2008, suffered a bit of nerve damage, recovered, and came home. Both Yabtsega and Mohammed now walk straight only because Berhanu needed a break.

Another boy, Teddy Legesse, fourteen years old, wasn't as lucky. He was brought to Rick by his uncle after his mother died of AIDS. She was a prostitute, and when Teddy was very small, it was his job to go out to buy condoms for her. Rick arranged for Teddy to have surgery, but there were complications. The boy became paralyzed and lost the use of his legs. His uncle holds Rick responsible, even though he'd signed off on the papers that fully explained the potential dangers if the boy had the surgery. The uncle was angry, accusatory, and difficult for Rick to deal with.

When I was there, Teddy was living at Mother Teresa's and getting physical therapy in the middle of a room where mentally defective kids were screaming. His uncle never visited. Eventually, the boy was moved to a chronic care facility where he was much happier and started school. He had friends and got regular physical therapy, and his neurologic function was returning. Despite numerous invitations, the uncle stayed away. Then one morning in December 2009, Teddy didn't wake up. He seems to have suffered a pulmonary embolism.

Rick wrote in an e-mail:

> *It is difficult to put this together medically.*
> *Sometimes we do not achieve success, but this*
> *should not discourage us from keeping on going.*
> *About sixty kids are in far better shape now,*
> *because of our efforts.*
> *I want to thank everyone who has helped*
> *Teddy over the past couple of years.*
> *Teddy, rest in peace.*

Rick sees patients in quick succession. There are so many of them lined up outside the clinic that Bayelign is sent to buy bunches of bananas to hand out to keep them going.

Benjamin Gorma, seventeen, is a back patient, but he had to be checked for heart and kidney problems as well. "They all go together," Rick explains. He turns to his laptop to review Benjamin's records and his x-rays, which he has digitized. (Rick's Ethiopian patients have the kind of electronic medical records that American health planners are still only dreaming about.)

The next patient is Tamrat Goza, age eighteen. His back is so deformed that it is up against the chest wall. His breathing capacity was at 15 percent, but it's improved with a simple plastic breathing machine.

Then came Radeit Joseph, a tiny two-year-old spine patient in a pink and yellow Polartec zip-up and red leggings with blue hearts. Rick says, "I'm working on getting her to Ghana or Los Angeles where there's a doctor who specializes in inserting growing rods." The toddler is crying, and Rick gets testy when he sees

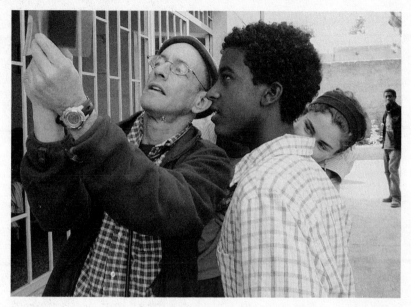

Rick in the garden at Mother Teresa's, examining an x-ray with Mesfin that will confirm his age.

that a cardiogram record is missing. "I shouldn't have to worry about these things," he snaps.

But the next minute, when Wubalem Desalign walks in, he returns to his gentle manner. He tells us she's seventeen and her name means "beautiful world." She's a back patient.

Sewalem, cured of Hodgkin's disease, returns to the clinic so Rick can see that his grossly distorted tumorous face has returned to a handsome normal. With medicines known as ABVD, purchased in India at a cost of $700 per patient, Rick says he regularly cures Hodgkin's disease.

Zelekia Tamam has had lifesaving surgery on her jaw by an American team that operated in the military hospital in Addis. "I actually traveled to America with a piece of her jawbone in my

187

suitcase," Rick tells us. "She had nice surgery, nice pathology. It wasn't cancer."

Binyam Mulugetta arrives wearing his school uniform. His parents report that he insists on going back to school despite Rick's order to stay home for at least two months following his back surgery in Ghana.

"I don't want him to be pushed or hurt," he tells them. "If the school needs a letter, we will send it. This is important; even if he has to repeat the year, it's better to have a healthy back for a lifetime."

Turning to Binyam, he says, "I'm the boss and you have to listen to me or I'll cut off your head, like a sheep. I have a knife in the car." The fifteen-year-old laughs.

Rick says the boy had "big, big surgery and needs time to heal." He tells the parents "if he wants to come to my house and see the other kids, that's fine. But no school."

The family found Rick by chance when they were passing the clinic on their way to get treatment for the boy's tonsillitis. Someone saw the boy's back and told them there was a doctor inside who could help. Rick tells the parents that the best spine doctor in the world operated on him. The grateful father said in his stilted schoolbook English, "God prepared you to help him and we wish God should watch over you and protect you." Then hesitantly, almost shyly, he asked if he might have a copy of the photographs of his son before and after surgery. Rick gave him the entire file, x-rays, CAT scans, and photos, all on a single CD.

"Ah, Elias Dingo Dima Dito Daya," Rick says, welcoming the next boy with the names of his father, grandfather, great-grandfather, and great-great-grandfather. Elias is checking in for his "allowance," and Rick couldn't be happier that he's there to take his money.

"He comes from a very poor family," Rick explains. "His mother is a widow with four kids who scrapes by by fetching water and washing clothes."

He is a good student, so Rick willingly pays his school tuition and gives him the equivalent of a dollar a day so he can get proper nutrition following his back surgery in Ghana. He tells Rick that he's eating two eggs a day and sometimes vegetables and an orange. Rick hands him 300 birr (about $30) for the month and tells him not to spend it all in one place.

"This is a fun day, isn't it," comments Rick as he moves on to the next patient.

Michael Endale comes in to be examined. He has chronic myelogenous leukemia that caused his spleen to expand. At one time it took up almost his entire stomach area. Now it is receding to normal size. "There is a drug that works on this disease," says Rick, "and I'm treating him with it. It is called Gleevec, which costs $70 a day, $2,000 a month. Here, it's free to poor people, but I had to prove the diagnosis, and proving it cost $450. Michael's mother is a widow and this is her only child, so I paid for the test."

Rick had to perform that test a couple of times because there were some false negatives. Then he contacted a pediatric oncologist at the University of Rochester, David Korones, who prescribed the proper dose for a child his size.

"He has too many white cells, and with that drug his kidney needs protection," Rick said, "I have the medicine (allopurinol) on the floor of my car and we can give it to him. He will have to

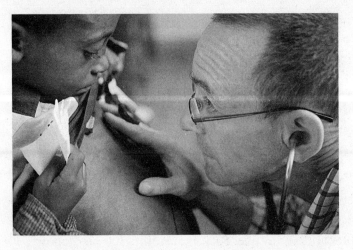

Michael Endale. Rick cured his chronic myelogenous leukemia with medi-cation that normally costs $70 a day. Rick arranged for them to be donated by Novartis.

take the medicine indefinitely. His spleen used to be over here," he says as he draws on the kid's trunk.

"Are you happy?" he asks Michael.

"Yes," says the boy.

Rick tells him he has a very good mother. "Some mothers abandon their kids here," he observes. She wants to take him back to their village for a week because she's run out of money, but Rick tells her that a lot of things could still go wrong, and they should move into Mother Teresa's.

Rick can slip quickly from charm, as with Jerusalem Tesfaye ("tell her she's more beautiful than last time") to impatience with the tears of nineteen-year-old Wolela Mohammed. She is com-plaining that she's been coming for some time and her family sent her away to live with prostitutes because they no longer be-lieve she's getting help.

"Tell her her back is not terrible. Some are much worse. I'm not the one who decides who gets surgery. It's the surgeons in America who decide. This is a social problem," Rick snaps. "I have to set limits."

Then he turns around on a dime to cheer up two people. He asks the translator to tell the next patient who arrives with her mother that she's a lucky girl. She looks like her beautiful mother.

Nadjia Kidere is the next patient, here on a first visit. She arrives wearing a long skirt, a scarf, and a purple blouse, which does not disguise the large lumbar hump on her back. She says she's sixteen, and when asked, she says she'd never been treated for TB. How had she heard about him? Rick asks her.

"Somebody around where I live told me there's a doctor who looks after this problem," she says. (Everybody goes to Rick's place!)

Her parents are dead, she has no brothers or sisters, and she works as a housemaid.

"Tell her I'm happy to have her as a patient," he says to Sister Fikerta, the nurse who is working with him on this day. "Tell her it's a good thing she came here. Maybe she can have an operation, maybe not, but in any case we can do things that can make her feel better."

He tells her he's going to send her for x-rays (he gives her money for that), but first he wants to take her picture. "Tell her she has to smile," he says.

Rick was thrilled last year when he read an article in the *Wall Street Journal* about the importance of these photographs. He sent the link around to everybody.

A study being presented Tuesday at a medical conference in Chicago suggests that radiologists should start examining something they usually ignore: the human face.

The eyes of modern radiology are so trained on high-tech images of arteries, organs, and bones that actual patients can become abstract concepts, rarely encountered in the flesh. But a study out of Israel found that including photographs of patients in their files enhanced radiologists' performance. "We recommend adding patient photographs as a routine protocol to the digital file of all radiographic examinations," the study concludes.

The director of Shaare Zedek hospital in Israel added, "When there is a picture, your attitude and approach changes—the human aspect is inserted."

"Who thought of this?" Rick said triumphantly, delighted that he now had the imprimatur of the entire medical community. "This isn't just a back . . ."

As he took her photograph, Nadjia Kidere told Rick she'd never spoken to a foreigner before.

"Tell her we're very ugly and very scary," Rick says.

"I'm not afraid," she replies.

Fikerta is laughing. "Dr. Rick is becoming funny," she says.

RICK HIMSELF GOT A HEARTY LAUGH out of one of the wonderful coincidences—or miracles—that seem to happen around him.

It involved a former patient, Desalegn Wanaw, now twenty-one, who was working as a welder at Mother Teresa's. He had left home when he was eight years old and severely crippled to live in Addis with an aunt who has since died. Four different times, his older brother Fentaye has come to Addis Ababa to look for him, and each time he was disappointed. He was beginning to believe his brother had died. On this particular Saturday, while I was there, Desalegn, wearing his blue denim work jacket, was walking up a street and suddenly saw his brother, whom he recognized from the tribal tattoos on his face, and called out to him. "No, you cannot be my brother," Fentaye said, fearing he was marked as a country rube and was about to be rolled by a big-city stranger. "My brother was crippled and stooped over," he said. "You are standing tall." Desalegn tried to convince him. He named their father and their mother, their sister, and their aunts. "You can't be my brother," Fentaye insisted, "my brother is crippled."

"Follow me," said Desalegn, "I'll show you." They walked to a quiet corner of the street, where Desalegn lifted his shirt and showed him the surgical scars on his back. "I met an American doctor named Rick and he flew me to a doctor in Ghana and now I'm a new boy," he explained. Fentaye could hardly believe that a boy who had been so deformed could now be so straight and strong and that in a city of more than four million people they had found each other on the same street. Rick was uplifted, ecstatic that yet another family had been reunited, and went around telling everyone the wonderful story.

This heartwarming tableau, however, soon shattered. The Sisters of Charity at Mother Teresa's expelled Desalegn some months later when he was found stealing from them. He not only stole from the sisters, he stole money from Rick—Rick who had sent him to Ghana for the fourteen-hour spine operation that had straightened his deformed back and made him whole, Rick who had taken money from his own contributions and paid the $10,000 needed to cover his travel and hospital expenses.

No good deed goes unpunished. (No, that's not from the Talmud.)

A year later, Desalegn turned up again at Mother Teresa's, where, with biblical forgiveness, they took him in. He was dressed in pajamas, had a shaved head, and was carrying a New Testament when he went up to Rick and attempted to kiss his feet. "I kept walking and said *layla gizeh,* 'some other time.' I will likely forgive him, but I don't want to make it easy for him."

To FINISH OFF HIS "FUN DAY," Rick headed for the chemo room where two little girls—not happy campers, as he says—were getting their intravenous medication. Next it was time to do a spinal tap on Aliyeh Mohammed, a nine-year-old orphan whose mother died in childbirth and whose father died in a construction accident. He came to Rick with a hugely disfiguring malignant tumor, which was diagnosed as Burkitt's lymphoma. The right side of his face had become a twisted and bulbous protruding mass that started at his jawline and dropped all the way down to his chest. Rick inserted an alarmingly long needle to remove spinal fluid and allow the infusion of chemotherapy to destroy the cancer cells. There is no hospital visit for this procedure.

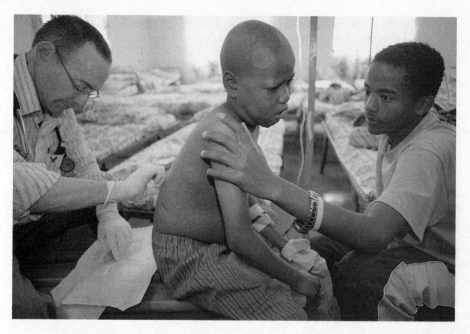

Time for Ali Mohammed's spinal tap. Teshale assists Rick to put the young patient at ease.

Ali Mohammed simply sits on his bed at the mission and Rick, assisted by one of the older boys from the house to provide assurance and perhaps hold a hand, does the spinal tap swiftly, as if it were no more than a simple injection. These kids never—and I mean never—cry out in pain. They barely wince when the needle goes in.

Jake Tabel, the visiting medical student who was working with Rick, said, "I remember when he would just sit on a patient's bed for a moment, or twirl them around in a dance, and for a brief moment nobody was sick anymore."

Rick was keeping up a running commentary as he loped through the mission grounds. He was saying that Ethiopians as a whole prefer injections to pills, believing that they are more effective.

"There is a cultural factor," Rick says. "Ethiopians *love* injections. There is a whole national cottage industry of illegal injectors who inject something (God knows what) for any malady. So by giving the injections (daily for the first two weeks and then twice weekly for the next six weeks), I was satisfying an important cultural need. They'd come for treatment because they loved injections, and then they would put up with having to swallow tablets as well."

He was explaining that he tries to limit himself to hearts, spines, and cancer, but he adds, "Whoever comes to me, I'll see what I can do to help."

Rick had asked Abel Ayalew, for example, to meet him this day at Mother Teresa's. He had news for him. Abel has been invited to study at the Colorado Center for the Blind in Littleton, and Rick wanted to help him get a student visa. The young man had been brought to the United States the year before to speak at the Hugh O'Brien Leadership Conference under the auspices of the Honolulu-based Ananda Foundation, which is also sponsoring him at the Littleton school.

Rick asked Abel to tell the story of how he'd gotten to Addis in the first place. "I came here by thief person," he replied. What he meant was that a kidnapper took him away from his home in the countryside and brought him to the capital to beg. He was four years old and sought after because little blind boys attract more money. Abel said the kidnapper, a modern-day Fagin, kept him and about ten or twelve other boys, gave them breakfast and a floor to sleep on, and sent them out each day to beg. At the end of each day he took the money the beggar children had collected. The kidnapper is an old man now and still sending kids out to beg. Abel says he knows where he is and vows that when he gets his visa for America, he will report him to the police. "Is he an evil man?" he was asked. "Yes, evil," he said in his very soft voice. "He's no angel."

Abel was a toddler when poisonous resin from a tree fell into his eyes and destroyed his sight. "Before I met you, it was a dark life for me," he tells Rick in a quiet, singsong voice, "and now it is light, and you have made life easy for me." He told us that a kind-hearted person he met on the street when he was begging took him into his home and taught him Braille and helped him attend a school for the blind. Abel can now make his own way around the city with the help of a cane. He is currently studying at the university in Addis and wants to become a history teacher. His only concern on this day was the weather in Colorado. "What's it like there?" he asked. It was then that Rick read him a letter he had just received from Abel's sponsors, who promised that he would be met at the airport with a heavy winter jacket.

RICK WILL PRETTY MUCH SEE anybody as long as nobody else is interested in him. On the first day of 2010, Rick took stock of his medical practice to date. He currently has 293 spine patients, having started with 3 in 2004. The majority of these patients were suffering from scoliosis and 39 percent had tuberculosis; 125 of them have had surgery. Rick is currently following 100 cardiac patients; 69 percent of them are suffering complications

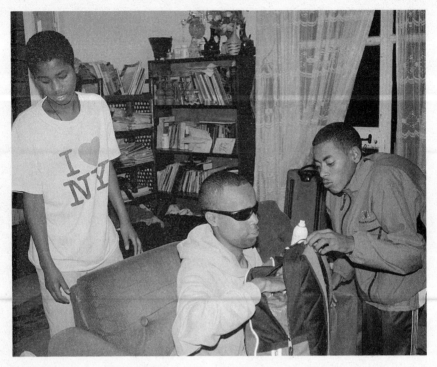

Abel preparing to leave for Colorado, at Rick's with Tesfaye and Melaku.

from rheumatic fever and 24 of them have had surgery. Among his cancer patients, he has sent 88 biopsies to the United States for analysis, treated 23 patients in Ethiopia, and treated some 50 Hodgkin's patients in the University Hospital.

HE'D BEEN DEALING FOR SOME TIME with a most unusual and unfortunate young woman who lived at Mother Teresa's, Merdya Abessa. It was painful even to look at Merdya. A grotesque tumor had pushed out the right side of her face a good eight inches, leaving an unseeing eye at the end. She walked around the mission with a shawl draped over her disfigurement. And she always smiled. Rick desperately wanted to help her and sent studies of her condition to as many doctors as he could think of. But he was getting no responses.

On one of his fund-raising visits to the States, Rick was in Minneapolis on a bitter cold day. He awoke with a start, then realized his alarm hadn't gone off and he was late. Grabbing his zippered bag with his prayer shawl and phylacteries, he figured he could say Shacharit, the traditional morning prayer, after he went to the meeting where he was expected. When he finished his talk, he asked his host whether there was a place he might go to pray.

"Go over there," the host said, pointing to an ultra-Orthodox synagogue, Bais Yisroyel. Upon finishing his prayers, Rick started chatting with a young man who happened to be there studying Talmud from the rabbi, a young man—as Rick's luck would have it—who turned out to be a neurosurgeon, Dr. Eric Nussbaum. The two doctors started talking about the kinds of cases they deal with, and Rick whipped out his laptop, which he'd brought in with him to protect it from the cold.

"Take a look at this one," he said.

Rick showed him a photograph of Merdya and explained that he'd looked everywhere, but no one would touch this case. Dr. Nussbaum was shocked; he'd never seen anything like it. But, he said, he thought he could help.

In January 2008, Rick went to the American consulate to get a visa for Merdya, another task he takes upon himself. It's not easy to get visas, particularly in the aftermath of 9/11, so Rick leaves plenty of time to work through the system. The consular official looked at the application and asked if Rick had a letter from the hospital that would treat Merdya.

"It's in my car," he said. "I'll get it."

The car has become Rick's mobile office, filled with papers, medication, and more than a little general detritus. By the time he returned to the visa window, a higher authority had been called in. Heather Guimond was the new deputy chief consul, and—here Rick's luck was again with him—she is the daughter of a doctor. Rick showed her Merdya's photographs, and Ms. Guimond responded immediately.

"I get this," she said. "My father is a neurosurgeon. Bring her in tomorrow, and we'll give her a visa."

It didn't hurt that Rick is at the top of the consulate's referral list for Americans needing medical help when in Ethiopia, and he gave his word that Merdya would return to Addis.

Some months later, Rick went with Merdya to Minneapolis. Rick travels so often that he's gotten to know the people at KLM, who warned him that if a patient looked too sick, he or she might not be permitted on the plane. Merdya's face was so alarmingly disfigured that Rick came up with the idea of buying her a chador that would cover her from head to toe, a costume that made the young woman dissolve in laughter when she saw herself in the mirror.

"It's been quite an adventure," Rick reported, "but we got Merdya from the mission to my home to Amsterdam to Ann Arbor and then to Minneapolis. Yesterday, she underwent an all-day surgery by a skull-based neurosurgeon, an oculo-plastic surgeon/neuro-ophthalmologist, and a cranio-facial surgeon. Her entire tumor was removed successfully. It was found to be 'fibrous dysplasia,' just fibroblasts. I asked a renowned neuropathologist if he had much experience with fibrous dysplasia. 'Nobody does,' he replied."

"What if my alarm had gone off on time," Rick says in wonder, positively exhilarated at the outcome. And that the chance meeting with Nussbaum occurred when he had gone to pray persuaded him once again of God's miraculous ways.

Nussbaum had gathered the team of doctors from around the region to assist in the surgery, and within a week of her arrival, Merdya had a reconstructed face and had started her recuperation while living in a home run by the Catholic church.

Before the surgery, the powers that be at Mother Teresa's in Addis had begun to suggest it was past time for Merdya to leave—after all, she was almost nineteen. Her friends there expressed their concern to Rick.

"Don't worry," he told them. "Merdya is under my protection. They won't throw her out."

But what was to become of her when she returned after the surgery? "She can go back to her village," he said, which leads me to wonder whether a conical *tukul* with a straw-thatched roof could contain this now-worldly woman who had learned how to find her way around Minneapolis on her own. "Or if she wants to open a kiosk, I'll help her," Rick said, "and if she wants to go to school, I'll send her. It's no use making somebody better if they can't have a life."

Before leaving for America, Merdya had talked of going to cooking school—tuition paid by Dr. Rick, of course—so she would have a trade, just like a former patient of Rick's who now cooks at Mother Teresa's and greets him like a beloved brother every time he enters the kitchen. It is there among the huge vats of steaming stew that Rick stops to eat an occasional breakfast consisting of ready-to-heat vegetarian meals left for him by Ethiopian Airlines personnel. He uncovers these delectable treats and, standing up, eats directly from the tinfoil without even bothering to warm them up.

Word of Dr. Nussbaum's willingness to help Merdya had become a small local sensation, and praise for Drs. Rick and Nussbaum soon came from a most unlikely source. Not long after reports of Merdya's surgery appeared in the local papers, Katie Baardseth, a pastor at the time at the Bethel Lutheran Church in Madison, Wisconsin (now a pastor at Midvale Lutheran Church in Madison), built her sermon of June 1, 2008, around the two Orthodox Jewish doctors and the teachings of Jesus—who Rick likes to point out is the third Jewish guy in the story.

Ms. Baardseth told her congregation:

> Hodes was deeply moved by Merdya's plight. He imme-
> diately began sending photos of her to brain specialists,
> asking if they could help. He contacted at least six world-
> renowned neurosurgeons. They all throw up their hands
> and say, "Oh my gosh, I've never seen anything like it."
> And that's it. That's like the end of the story. Hodes said,
> "It was very frustrating for me, knowing we could po-
> tentially save her life. But it was a great challenge be-
> cause nobody was interested in helping her."

Pastor Baardseth continued,

> During a fund-raising trip to Minneapolis last Novem-
> ber, Hodes said, God led him to a doctor who could
> help Merdya. . . . Dr. Nussbaum was willing to attempt
> what many other doctors had declined to do. . . . He
> said one sentence that nobody else had said. Unlike the

other six surgeons, Nussbaum added, "I'd love to try to help this lady."

The story of Hodes' quest to save the young girl from Ethiopia is much like what Jesus is telling us in today's gospel. . . . Hodes' requests for help to doctors were met with sympathy when they said, "Oh my gosh, I've never seen anything like that." But those doctors were only hearers and not doers. When Hodes showed Nussbaum the photos of the . . . girl's tumor he heard his fellow doctor say the words that mattered—"I'd love to try to help." In other words, "I'm not just going to listen to your story; I'm going to do something about it."

"Build your house on the rock when you hear about someone's problem and you respond to it. Build your house on the rock when you not only hear the word of Jesus, but you do it."

All of this, it would seem, is one of those heartwarming fairy tales come true, but not quite. Merdya was developing another idea. She decided that she liked it in America and didn't want to go back; she wanted to request "political asylum." Rick was infuriated. He'd given his word to the American consulate that she would not overstay her medical visa, and a failure to return would compromise his future efforts to help other patients.

Rick tried to contact the organization that had arranged for Merdya's housing, but got no answer. He still hopes to pursue the matter. Meanwhile, Merdya is in the United States. She's gone underground.

Once again, no good deed goes unpunished.

NO USE TAKING A PICTURE
OF A SKELETON

WHEN ELEVEN-YEAR-OLD ATSEDE—the girl Rick calls Miss Ethi-opia—eventually went to Los Angeles in 2008 for cardiac surgery, she too got a taste for America. The Mending Kids program set her up with a family in Malibu, California, where she could live in a real home for the first time in her life. By the time she returned to Addis in December, she was a healthy girl wearing a sequin-decorated, bell-bottom pink warm-up suit and Converse sneakers. She also had with her four suitcases filled with a wardrobe for a Malibu princess (including UGG shearling boots to wear in a city where the temperature almost never goes below fifty degrees). Atsede insisted on leaving all the suitcases at Rick's. She pointed to each one and said, "No mission," knowing that if she brought all her finery to Mother Teresa's, it would be distributed to other kids.

She proudly carried a book of photographs that her host family had put together for her: Atsede at Disneyland, Atsede in pink tulle in a dance recital, Atsede at the beach, Atsede in the private swimming pool, Atsede at Thanksgiving dinner. As she showed her mother the album, people at the mission gathered around and looked at the photographs with astonishment.

This was a world beyond their imagination. Her mother told us that Atsede's father had gone to prison for killing a man and

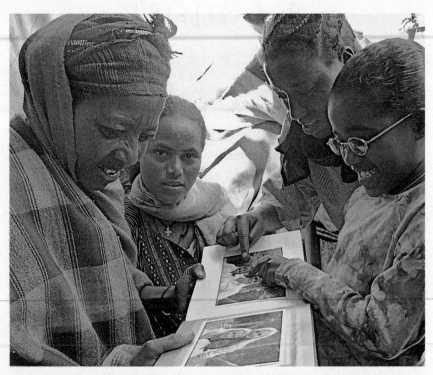

Atsede introduces her friends at Mother Teresa's to life in America, a world beyond their imaginations.

some time after that she and her daughter ended up at Mother Teresa's. She kept saying over and over again that she thanks God for Rick. Holding her hands to her heart and looking toward the heavens, she prayed that Rick would live forever.

Atsede's ailing mother began asking Rick to let her daughter live at his house, but for now at least he has decided to leave her where she is. "I considered having her at home," he said, "but it's a lousy idea and pattern: send a kid to USA, get them spoiled, move into my home, and I have to raise them when they have loving parents somewhere else."

One foster parent pointed out that it's difficult to avoid what he called "a case of the gimmes" when these children come to America. Workineh, the boy with Ollier's disease, which made his hand look like a medieval mace, was accepted for a series of surgeries at Cedars-Sinai in Los Angeles. Rick is convinced he was the most difficult hand patient in the United States.

At Christmastime his foster family told Rick, "He is infected with the 'I want' syndrome that the rest of us have this time of year. It's hard to know why you shouldn't ask for the moon if you've been given everything else you've ever dreamed of in life. His latest request is a golf cart for his next birthday, 'Me car, my birthday.' He's learning a bit of English and also campaigning to go to school. As the neighborhood kids leave each morning, he asks, 'Me school?' He is somewhat appeased with his weekly tutor and our trips to the library and museum. He's got an active mind and a winsome personality."

And Workineh also tried every stratagem he could think of to stay in America—including a request that his father be tested for AIDS. But now he's back home, and father and son are happy.

Even Rick's own son, the sensible Dejene, wrote the following in an e-mail after less than a term at a school in Ohio when his written English still needed work:

> *Hey dad*
> *i have been thinking about my computer and i do not think i need it now if it costs that much may be in a few years but i do not raly need one right now.*
>
> *but what i do need is some thing that i can use for music so a lot of my friends just got the new ipod that just came out and it is very nice and it is just 240 for every thing. if you are ok with it can you place try to get it for me and because you are like a teacher you all so get discounts so place look in to it for me. and if you want to do a deal like me working for you during the summer so that i can pay you back we can also do that. think about it and tell me. it is an ipod touch 8gb. i have used it some times from my friends and it is rely nice. Tell me what you think.*

And here's what Rick—who keeps his kids on an extraordinarily tight budget—replied:

> *Dejene my baby,*
> *Thanks so much for your e-mail. In some way, it shows that I am succeeding as a parent, albeit a financially poor one.*
> *I could give you a short answer in Hodes language: 'KD' (Keep Dreaming).*

Or I could give you a long answer: study hard,
get great grades and pray that I win the lottery.

Love, Dad

Rick had more serious matters to worry about, chief among them, a young boy who was weighing heavily on his mind and his heart. He checked on him every day in his dormitory at Mother Teresa's, praying for another miracle that might save him.

Redai had come to Rick's clinic three years earlier with severe abdominal pain that was eventually diagnosed as IPSID, immunoproliferative small intestinal disease, which, if treated, has only a one-third chance of remission. Untreated, it is fatal. Rick consulted with a number of doctors in the United States, and a top expert from Harvard recommended a particular course of chemotherapy. Redai, at sixteen, was a high school senior, spectrally thin with an extraordinarily beautiful chiseled face. He was unusually articulate, spoke and wrote excellent English, and continued to drag himself to school even though he had decided he would rather die than continue suffering. He took the first rounds of chemotherapy but was refusing the last two. He kept saying he did not want to be saved. He did not want pills or even the injections in which Ethiopians place so much faith.

Redai occasionally helped out at the clinic, where he had a remarkably gentle manner with the patients. One day he was translating for Rick when I raised my camera to photograph a patient. He held up his hand to stop me, thinking I was taking a picture of him.

Later, very politely, he asked to speak to me outside.

"I'm sorry that I was rude," he said, "but there's no use taking a picture of a skeleton."

This gave me the opportunity to add my plea that he accept the final two rounds of chemo. I told him I had seen him with the clinic patients and thought he would make a fine (and very handsome) doctor and that if he didn't make every effort to get better, it would be a great loss not only for his friends but for the country, which so desperately needs people like him. I told him he had better physicians treating him than most people get even in America and that he should give it a chance.

I thought I might be getting through to him, but he abruptly ended our conversation by saying he wouldn't do it. I asked him if he'd see me the next day at the clinic. No, he said, but I could come to see him in the dormitory.

Sister Brigitta, then the chief nurse at the mission, had been trying and trying to convince Redai to continue the treatment. She appealed to his strong spiritual convictions.

"Negative thoughts are not God's way," she told him while sitting on the side of his bed. "We are all in the hands of God, you can't see the progress because your cancer is inside; go to the chapel and find out what God has for you."

And Rick too had tried repeatedly, but Redai lay on his cot with the covers over his face, refusing to eat and refusing medication. "I've had treatment, and I've eaten, and I see no physical or health changes," Redai explained.

Rick used his most gentle tone when they spoke: "We say in America that it's always darkest before the dawn and you're in the tunnel and can't see the light so you have to keep going forward. . . . You have a complicated and unusual disease but not at all the worst we have here. You have very good doctors, you have me, working the best I can to help you, and you have the doctors at Harvard. You have a good shot, do you believe me?

Why would I lie to you and spend money and work so hard if I didn't think you had a shot. You know I'm a lazy guy. You know, did you ever play cards? Well, when you play cards, you have to play with those you are dealt even if they're not the ones you wanted."

About a month earlier, Redai told Rick that if he really loved him, he would get him an iPod and an Obama T-shirt! Later Redai said he was just kidding, but Rick wasn't so sure.

Redai had also written a lengthy letter to Monica Woll, the JDC volunteer who had been trying to encourage him. He tried to explain himself.

> *Now and for the future I don't want to take the chemo b/c I don't have any hope to be alive in this world for the future. I have known about my disease. . . . my disease couldn't be kill b/c of the medicine so I don't want to suffer b/c of the medicine. . . . I was eating different kinds of foods; I was eating fish and chocolate always except yesterday and today, but I don't have any physical and health change. So what is the function of needing special foods for me? It is useless! So I think it is better to save the money instead of wasting it for useless. . . . I don't have the probability to be alive so it is better to die instead of suffering.*

A week later, he agreed to one more round of chemo, and everyone breathed a sigh of relief.

"Then we will see," he said.

Rick promised to make the treatment as easy as possible for

him. He would sit with Redai throughout the entire session and would provide a lot of antinausea medicine. Redai's next request was for a Snickers bars, and a week later he told Monica that she needn't bother visiting him unless she brought *dorowat* (chicken stew) from a particular restaurant.

That was the last straw for Rick. It was time to have a serious conversation with Redai, time to let the boy know that Rick and his staff were not his waiters!

A month later, Rick reported that Redai was looking worse than ever. "I told myself that he cannot get any thinner, he looks like a thin veneer of brown skin stretched over his skull bones, his eyes totally sunken back, zygomatic arch protruding like an oversize speed bump on a smooth road."

On several occasions Rick left home at 7:00 A.M. to see if Redai had made it through the night. Rick said, "If he was going to die, I needed to say something substantial to him. . . . I sat with him and held his hand. I didn't want him to give up so I chose my words carefully. I recalled hearing Elie Wiesel tell physicians at the Mayo Clinic, 'you should never make the patient give up hope.' And I considered what the Talmud says of this situation:

"They who visit the sick should speak with judgment and tact; they should speak in such a manner so as neither to encourage false hopes, nor to depress by words of despair.

"I sat on a chair next to him and took his left hand into my hands. 'Redai,' I said with tears in my eyes, 'it's hard to understand what's going on here. I cannot fathom how God runs the world, and frankly, I cannot understand a world where kids like you suffer. It's not my design. But I don't think anyone else in this country would have put in the time to come up with the diagnosis or figure out what to do about it.

"'Now you're not doing well. But I can see you're a fighter. Until recently, you were still going to school. You even made us arrange your chemotherapy around your exam schedule.'"

Rick feared these were the last words he would say to him, and he knew it wasn't the time to mention that Redai had been "a manipulative teenage jerk" when he demanded the Obama T-shirt or special chicken dinners.

"Redai," Rick continued, "listen. It has been my privilege to be your doctor. It has not been easy, and sometimes you have not been easy. But I want you to know how much I care about you and how much I want you to get better. I pray for you—three times a day, actually."

Redai nodded, and Rick kept talking: "And now, what can I say? Who knows what will happen? Who knows what will happen to you, or to me, or to your mom in the next day or two? We are all in God's hands, and God loves you. It's tough to make sense of all of this. If I were running the universe, I wouldn't give bad diseases to kids, that's for sure.

"But God runs the world, I tell myself over and over, and we pick up the pieces. Redai, God is watching over you and caring for you."

Rick sat holding Redai's hand for the next twenty minutes as he breathed audibly. His pulse was surprisingly strong.

Later that day, one of the mission volunteers, a German medical student, came by. "Dr. Rick, I see you praying with Redai. What do you pray for? Do you pray that God takes him swiftly and painlessly?"

"Good question," Rick replied. "I've given it a lot of thought.

In this case, he is a teenage boy with cancer. I want him to be cured, so that's what I pray for. If God wants him to have a good death, God will give him a good death. But my job is to heal my patients, so I am praying for a good life, not a swift death."

Rick then stopped two of the nuns and put the same question to them. They agreed completely with the answer he had given the German student. A nun from Burundi told him, "Dr. Rick, we do what we can, and we then leave it up to God. You have done your job, and you can sleep soundly knowing that."

Redai's cheerful, bright-eyed mother had come to the mission to be with him. Her hair was braided in tight rows, and over her black dress she wore a bright yellow T-shirt bearing a message written in French. She scurried around in her plastic sandals doing what she could to help and feed her son.

"I am told," said Rick, "that she understands how close he is to death. This is her only child in the world. In America, this intelligent woman could easily be a third-grade teacher. Here, she is an illiterate peasant woman who was found by the nuns scrounging for food in a garbage dump in Tigrai. They offered to send Redai to a Catholic school, to feed him and educate him. He was bright, he was motivated, and quickly learned English."

One evening Rick told himself that the boy couldn't last the night. "With trepidation, I came early Thursday morning, and he actually looked significantly better, his eyes less sunken, and he asked for juice. I could not explain his change."

"It is difficult for me to accept his impending death," Rick said to me at the time, "and I have a fantasy that he'll get better."

Then Rick received a call on his home phone at 9:00 A.M. as he worked on his laptop in the living room. It was from a gastroenterologist at Cornell Medical School who wanted Rick's help with a relative of hers. Rick took this opportunity to ask about her practice and kept her on the phone—it was 1:00 A.M. in New York—to talk about the various intestinal diseases she treated. He told her about Redai.

"I have a kid with IPSID who's not doing well," he said. "Any suggestions?"

"You want to try rifaximin," she replied. "I probably have some lying around. How can I get it to you?"

One of the mission volunteers was back in the States so Rick asked her to FedEx it to the young man so he could carry it back. Rick had heard of this drug but had never used it; he decided it was worth a try. He figured "nothing is going to hurt at this point."

The recommended dose is one tablet three times a day, but that's for an American of about 170 pounds. Rick decided to cut the pills in half because Redai weighed only 48 pounds. He took out his Swiss Army Knife—"all our kitchen knives are dull as a froe," he explained—bisected a bunch of the pills and started Redai on rifaximin, half a tablet three times daily. He added half a tablet of azithromycin, which he keeps on hand for the trachoma patients in Lalibela.

Redai was declining, but Rick held on to every positive sign, allowing his fantasy to flourish. Every day after clinic, he stopped in to see Redai and sat with him for ten or fifteen minutes, holding his hand and praying, chatting with him intermittently.

"The other day he asked for some bottled juice," Rick remembered, "and I ran out and got him a box of apple and a box of mango with a straw to perforate the small round foil opening."

The next day Rick was astounded—and even hopeful—when Redai asked for yogurt.

"Could you get me some?"

"What kind," Rick said.

"Just plain."

"I did not want to leave my car alone on the street, so I asked a volunteer to drive down the hill with me to two small grocery stores with refrigerators who would stock yogurt. He readily agreed. We gave him the yogurt, and I said good-bye."

Rick went home for a couple of hours and returned to bring a few more doses of medicine for Redai. "He was sitting up, and I asked how he's doing. 'I'm depressed,' he said. 'I hate this IV.' 'I understand,' I said, 'it can't be easy. What can I get you?'"

"Yogurt," he said.

"Redai, we got you yogurt a few hours ago," Rick said.

"Yeah, I finished it," he said. "He had eaten a half liter of yogurt, and then wanted more.

"'With pleasure,' I said, wondering whom I could get to fetch the yogurt while I stayed in my car, which had my camera and computer.

"I went to the small volunteer house on the compound, which was locked. I then looked around—nobody to be seen. I then went into the chapel, where the nuns were sitting on the ground in front, and a few scattered volunteers were behind. I approached an old Irish fellow and tapped him on the shoulder. 'Can you help me?' I asked. 'Right now?' he said. 'Yeah, immediately.'"

They stepped outside, and Rick explained to him that Redai was a sixteen-year-old dying of cancer who wanted yogurt and that he needed someone to run into the grocery store while he waited in his car. The man agreed immediately. Rick recalled,

"I did not know him except to say hi. He looks to be about a 74-year-old Irishman. I imagined him to be a quiet, antiquarian bookseller. I asked him what he does. 'I am retired for twelve years,' he said, 'but I was a one-man band.' He lives in rural Ireland, goes into town for church services but that's it. I assumed he was a devout Catholic.

"Wrong again; turns out that he's a Christian Scientist. As we drove down to Arat Kilo, he told me that he was very athletic in his early 20s and then developed a lot of orthopedic problems and dislocations of joints. He said that a friend introduced him to Christian Science, he prayed, and he was healed. 'That was it,' he said. 'Enough of medicine. Now I work on love. I feed the retarded kids and hold their hands. It works.'

"'Sorry to get you out of church,' I said.

"'Doctor Rick,' he said, in his careful Irish diction, 'how can I sit and pray when I can be helping a dying boy? God does not want to keep us locked up in churches. Some of the best Christians I know—far better than myself—refuse on principle to go to church and are much better people. God wants us out in the world. This is what I should be doing. Thank *you* for asking for my help.' We drove down the hill, and I waited while he got two containers of yogurt.

"When I came in today, Redai was sitting on his bed, his mom spooning him ravioli.

"I began to wonder if this phone call from a stranger in New York City could end up saving Redai's life, using a drug I'd hardly heard of. It's a wonderfully appealing idea to my fantasy system.

"In the meantime, Redai sits up and eats yogurt, still gravely ill, but one tiny step in the right direction.

"Realistically, it is highly unlikely that he'll live another week. I realize that. He is one of numerous items to pay attention to on my daily to-do lists that I write on white index cards every morning. I really can't sit with him for hours and get anything else done—like a government report, like my son's financial aid forms, like U.S. taxes, like getting patients to India in the coming weeks. So I go in twice a day and sit, hold hands, and pray."

About a week later, Rick left for a visit to the United States. The call came on Friday, March 13. Redai had died. His body was wrapped in white muslin and placed in a special room with other wrapped bodies to be picked up by a city truck that calls at the mission once a day.

"It's part of the job," Rick said tearfully. "I'm grateful that we could give him a shot at life and at least a year of better life; at least we gave him a chance. I'll say a prayer for him today," he said. "It's a tough thing to make sense of. . . . I recall an episode of the TV show *M*A*S*H* where [as he remembers it] Hawkeye says, 'I never get used to it. I always feel there was something more I should have done.'

"Honeycutt says, 'But, Hawk, you did everything that was humanly possible.'

"'I know how it's supposed to go,' Hawkeye continues, 'shock, anger, readjustment . . . but all we ever see is the shock and anger.'

"'Hawk,' Honeycutt continues, 'look what you're doing—you're punishing yourself with guilt.'

"'I think I'm having an identity crisis,' Hawkeye says. 'I know I'm Dr. Pierce, but I want to be God.'

"Honeycutt looks up and comments: 'If you ever get the job, don't forget your old friends.'"

11

I'M HERE AND THEY'RE NOT

SEMEGNEW, RICK'S OLDEST ADOPTED SON, WAS at school in Ohio in 2007 when he saw that CNN was running a contest called "Name Your Hero." He was certain he knew just the right person. Semegnew is shy and soft-spoken by nature, perhaps because of a severe childhood and possibly because he is troubled by his short stature. His back surgery left him at four feet, seven inches.

But there was nothing shy about the letter he sent to CNN:

> *The greatest hero I have ever known in my life*
> *is My Dad. I am not sure if hero is the right word*
> *to describe My Dad. . . . I think I might instead*
> *call him the savior of the world, mostly Africans.*
> *A lot of people call him Father Teresa. My Dad*

has saved the lives of hundreds of Africans. Besides the five adopted sons there are also seventeen other kids who are living in one of his two houses. The number of kids in our house is never stable—not because someone dies, but because we always have newcomers. My dad e-mailed me last week saying he has two more new kids who have no one to support them and need medical attention . . .

Semegnew went on to tell the story of how Rick cured him and changed his life as well as the lives of the many kids who are treated in three different clinics in Ethiopia. He wrote:

I greatly admire what My Dad does, but I feel bad for him because I have seen how doctors live in America, and even in Africa. They have beautiful homes, but my dad does not. The only thing he cares about is the number of patients he is saving every day. He does not have enough time to eat and eats in his car driving to work, and he does not have enough time to sleep, either. I hope some day he will realize that he is pushing himself too much. He needs to take a little time to relax. I love him and love what he does, but it is too much. Thank you for giving me a chance to write about My Hero—My Dad.

Semegnew Hodes

Out of seven thousand submissions, this letter from a foreign student in Barnsville, Ohio, who had no influence in the media or anywhere else so impressed the judges that Rick became one of three finalists from around the world. First place went to a man who runs a missionary school in Kenya, but the network gave Rick $10,000 as the first runner-up.

"That's one back surgery," said Rick, using his measure for just about everything.

Even after two decades in Africa, Rick continues to find genuine excitement where most others find nothing but pain and misery, and now he was beginning to get some recognition for treating the sickest of the sick, the people others had given up on.

He thinks nothing of hopping on a transatlantic flight as he did to come to New York for the CNN award ceremony. For those of us who consider any air travel a contemporary circle of hell, Rick proves himself a true eccentric when he declares, "I love airports." He actually finds them restful. He settles down in a lounge, has a drink, and casts himself adrift in the Internet. This is the best time, when you know he's making a plane connection, to reach him by e-mail—normally not an easy thing.

Full of nervous energy, he stays extraordinarily trim, never allowing his weight to go over 128 pounds; he likes to say that his body is genetically engineered to fly coach! When he's lucky and the flight isn't full, he gets to stretch out for the night on three seats, creating what he calls "poor man's first class."

By design, his travel routes tend to be maddeningly circuitous, hardly what one would expect from a geography major. He may be the only person who travels through Atlanta to get from Memphis to Cleveland just so he can add frequent flier miles, which he uses to send kids for medical help.

One time his flight was delayed for many hours, and the airline gave each passenger a coupon that could be ex-

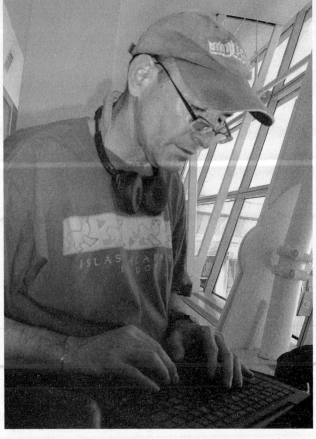

Rick roaming the Internet at the airport, one of his favorite places to relax.

changed for food in the terminal's restaurants. Rick organized the other passengers and persuaded them to give their coupons to the janitorial staff, who all seemed to be West Africans.

"I gave a woman with a broom a $10 coupon, and she nearly kissed me," Rick said. "The restaurant staff raised their eyebrows as the janitors stood in lines and paid in vouchers."

Rick is such an anomaly in this world and so devoid of sanctimony that it's perplexing that he sometimes seems so normal. He likes good conversation or a good joke, and he relishes whatever inside-the-Beltway political gossip he can pick up. He avidly monitors the news of the world on his battered laptop, and he always wants to know what people are saying about the likes of Henry Kissinger and President Obama and the Clintons.

He was terribly pleased with himself recently when he got hold of a piece of inside information about who was to be appointed the next chief of USAID (the U.S. Agency for International Development) long before folks in Washington knew it. "Here I was in Addis Ababa, and I knew something they didn't," he crowed.

It is impossible not to notice that amid all the misery he sees, Rick is having a hell of a time with his life. He enjoys each day, a phenomenon that is common among people who are in the business of doing good. Peter Singer, the Princeton ethicist, in his book *Ethics into Action,* saw this very same thing in Henry Spira, who is credited with initiating the successful animal rights movement. Spira seemed to Singer a most happy man. When Rick saw Mother Teresa and her acolytes the first time, he remarked on how serene and happy they were.

Maybe it's the joy of a life well lived, the satisfaction of a compassionate life. "Meaning," Rick has said, "is the only thing that matters. It gives us happiness, and it gives us a feeling of worth."

However happy Rick may be, he has been known to drive those around him crazy. He abhors routine and avoids it no matter what the price, which may be why he leads the life he does. It is a life in which he can be unpredictable and get away with it. He hates to make plans, he is chronically late, and he does only what he chooses to do.

Rick is fortunate that he's able to captivate eager volunteers who come to help him and sometimes stay for months at a time. Chloe Malle, for one, came with me to Addis on my first trip during her Christmas break from Brown University. She was walking with me on Arat Kilo the day I found Danny, and during her visit, she was so overwhelmed by the good work Rick was doing she decided to return after graduation to work with him for almost a year. She was already an old hand in the third world, having worked in southern India one summer for Smile-Train, an experience that prepared her to deal with some of the most difficult cases in Rick's clinic. She was compassionate and gentle with patients who were often hard to even look at, and she made herself useful in innumerable ways. Among other things, she was put in charge of the critical breathing tests Rick needs for most of his patients. She also did what she could for Redai.

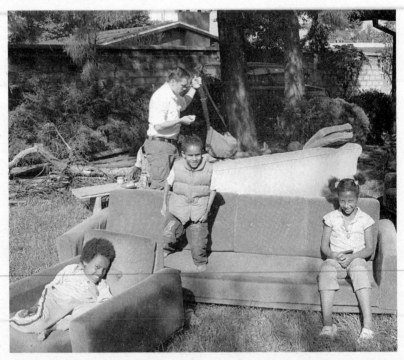

Kids in plein air enjoying the outdoor living room during Chloe's renovation of the house.

At Rick's house, she got the kids off to school in the mornings, tutored them, and attended their parent-teacher meetings. She also took on additional chores that Rick had no time and no desire to do himself, like bringing order to the almost indecipherable financial accounts and to the house itself, which, although Rick never noticed it, had become dingy and frayed from so many kids tramping through it.

She was determined to get rid of the grunge that had built up in a house with twenty kids living there—to say nothing of Rick's own pack-rat tendencies. She did away with the stained couches and upholstered chairs and brought in a new décor with crisp plaid autumn-hued curtains. Bookcases were organized and x-rays and reports were put in order and moved to the JDC office—although a great number still remained in jagged piles in Rick's room and the bathtub, his unique filing cabinet.

Some time later, when Rick was on a trip to the United States, Chloe decided to attack his bedroom, a task that turned out to be considerably more daunting than Hercules's labor of cleaning out the Augean stables. Although this room, unlike those of ancient myth, contained no detritus from animals, it did have an accumulation of many years with many strata, and the job lasted much longer than one day.

Once Chloe got permission to enter this sanctum sanctorum, she discovered a veritable archaeological dig. On just her first pass at the job, she unearthed artifacts that provided some excellent clues for the study of Rick Hodes.

Among the treasures, first of all, was the food, which he seems to bring home from everywhere he travels, great quantities of tea and candied ginger and nuts that he has squirreled away and apparently forgotten. Chloe took what was still edible and made a food chest, dividing it into sweet and savory. There were also medicines of all kinds, much of it expired, tucked in among the x-rays and files. Postcards and dozens of yellowing Rosh Hashanah cards provided evidence of his many friends; bills told of his expenses; and fifteen different bathing suits and broken swim goggles attested to his chosen form of exercise. There was also a lady's bra left on a hanger in the closet some years before that told of—all right, let's not go there. Chloe also found fifteen ties, four of them with an elephant motif, suggesting that he might be a Republican—but this would be entirely misleading. There were many pairs of the same brown shoes he buys over and over again, but he still holds on to the old worn-out ones, and the duffels full of white tube socks that he regularly brings back from the States but that the evidence suggests he was probably too tired to distribute when he got home. And for anyone seeking enlightenment about his reading preferences, she found a trove worthy of the Collyer brothers of back copies of *The New Yorker, The Economist,* and the *New England Journal of Medicine* as well as a juggling kit and a recorder.

One or two artifacts survived the renovation: the battered wooden table that sits in the dining area and serves as desk, card table, ironing board, and x-ray viewer stand is still surrounded by four rickety chairs and one backless perch that looks like an invitation to an accident. Chloe refitted the servants' quarters in the back as bedrooms—with real beds for the kids. Eventually, Rick agreed to rent an auxiliary house—which Chloe also fixed up, even constructing by hand beds for the kids who would live there—and filled it with the teenage boys who no longer had any elbow room in the main house. That left Rick with only nine or ten at home—and it's an easy guess what that might mean.

"I think he'll fill up the house again," says Addisu. "When we were only four or five, he said 'no more.' But he's a very warm-hearted guy. If he sees somebody he likes and he can help, he's not going to say 'I'm not going to help this kid.'"

All of these kids have pretty much won the lottery in a country where hopelessness lives side by side with unrelenting poverty made worse by unspeakable disease. At Rick's they are in Ethiopian heaven where they are protected and fed and schooled. But like any house full of kids it can become a madhouse.

One afternoon during a bout of roughhousing, one of the boys said to another, "You can't beat me up because I'm Rick's kid." Rick quickly assured the first boy that he could beat up anyone he wants. But it is true that the adopted children have become an elite within this group, and not only because they get taken out for Chinese food every Sunday night!

When Addisu Hodes is in Addis, he refuses to join the group because he thinks it's unfair to the others. Mesfin Hodes—whose name means "Duke" and who loves to wear the caps and sweatshirts from the university in North Carolina that bears his name—has no such compunction and even feels he deserves every privilege and more.

I would have thought these kids would be filled with gratitude considering what might have happened to them. Wrong. Mesfin, the youngest adopted boy who is being treated for a growth hormone deficiency, has a litany of complaints and, in his very good English, is not at all reticent about airing them: Rick spends too much time with his patients and too much money on them. He spends too little time—and definitely too little money—on his own kids.

But where would Mesfin be if it weren't for Rick?

"Somebody else would have adopted me," he says petulantly, completely ignoring the fact that when Rick found him he had been placed with the nonadoptable children at Mother Teresa's.

Rick manages a wry smile and says only, "Mesfin is king of the house."

Or maybe an emperor, like Haile Selassie, who was willful, spoiled, and haughty. Mesfin sometimes strikes me as a case study in how even an orphan boy in Addis can become a spoiled child.

One day early on in my first visit, I found him lounging on the sofa, having skipped school because he said he wasn't feeling well. His sense of entitlement is such that when the kids got rooms and beds after the Chloe makeover, he demanded a private room. He finally agreed to share with a roommate, but only after a lot of kicking and pouting.

He complains that he's bored, and not only when he's sick.

"There's nothing to do but just sit around," he says.

He wishes to be amused. He wants a foosball and/or a Ping-Pong table. To this, Rick says "KD"—keep dreaming, the Hodes mantra.

Rick seems to have infinite patience when it comes to his kids and says that all he needs to do is hold his breath until the teenage gimmies end. But, he observes dryly, "How quickly they forget that they are alive!" He also keeps his sense of irony: *Why did God ask Abraham to sacrifice his son Isaac when he was twelve years old? Because if he were thirteen, it wouldn't be a sacrifice.*

Rick's equanimity is not easily shattered. "We all get mixed reviews," he once observed. "I met a reporter who spent ten days with Albert Schweitzer and could not stand him. One of the people who spent time with me here rarely speaks with me now (and I didn't even make a pass at her). The very religious mother of a former volunteer (who apparently did not appreciate my sense of humor) told her son I'm 'sick' and to never hang out with me again. I won't try to defend myself . . . except to say I'm here and they're not."

Anyway, he takes considerable comfort from commentaries on the Torah:

> *A person who takes an orphan into his home is like the father of a child: He gives life and sustains him.*
> *Who performs tzedakah all the time?: A person who brings an orphan into this home. He is always doing tzedakah, this is the top level. [Tzedakah is loosely translated as "charity" but encompasses the idea of justice and fairness.]*

Rick's children are not quick to express their gratitude to him, so an e-mail from Addisu was particularly cherished:

> *It seems like I only e-mail you when I want you to do something for me. Consequently, I thought I would send an e-mail to tell you how much you have affected my life. You are the one who had made me the person I am today. You know, those who know me real well and know where I'm coming from, they congratulate me because of my experience but really it shouldn't be me who should be congratulated, I just walked through an open door that was opened by you. Hence, you should be congratulated for taking the effort to open the door so it would be simple for me to walk through*

it and be the person I am today. If it wasn't for
you, simple things such as knowing soccer existed
would have never crossed my head let alone to
grow up playing it and be the captain of my high
school team and be considered the best player at the
school. There are more but I think you get the point
and I don't need to mention everything.

The kids in Rick's house have to realize how fortunate they are—even Mesfin when he's not in one of his moods. Mostly, they do not forget what they were rescued from, even if occasionally they learn—as do all kids—that there is more out there to wish for.

As Rick says, "There's them, and then there's everybody else in Ethiopia."

The older boys definitely realized how lucky they were when Rick told them he had decided to close the second house; it was time for them to look after themselves. He would help pay rent for some of them, but those with jobs would have to take responsibility for their own housing.

The house the boys had been living in cost 9,000 birr or about $900 a month, and with the lease up and the rent about to be increased, Rick felt he had supported the older boys long enough. Three of the boys who had finished their education and had jobs, he decreed, should be on their own. Endale agreed, saying (in a surprisingly Western form of psycho-speak) that the older boys had become "addicted to dependency."

Rick dropped this bombshell at a meeting with the boys one night after Shabbat services, and the next day he left for the United

States. The boys sat there in silence and shock. Bewoket walked in toward the end of the meeting and asked, "Who died?"

The boys naturally turned to Chloe, who decided to use tough love on them. She would not go house hunting for them. They had to do it themselves.

So they started looking—and squabbling: one house was too far from the bus, another was too small, and yet another required too much rent in advance. Now, with the help of an American benefactor—a doctor in Atlanta who knows some of the boys—they've settled into a place that is even more cramped than they are accustomed to, but at least the ten of them can remain together.

One day, three of the boys, Solomon, Teshale, and Mohammed, came to Chloe's house to review their vocabulary words for that week's quiz, but it soon became apparent that they had come to watch a movie on her laptop. Mohammed had brought a pirated Charlie Chaplin DVD housed in a makeshift envelope of worn printer paper that had a pixilated image of Charlie with his bowler and mustache underneath the title, *The Bast of Charlie Chaplin*.

"I was hesitant to put this excuse for a DVD in my computer," Chloe said, "but Mamo's eagerness overruled any concerns I had, and I moved my hand away from the CD slot like raising a drawbridge. Fortunately for my hard drive, it was not the correct DVD format."

Solomon picked up a hair dryer that Arielle, an American friend, had left in the living room.

"He looked at the hair dryer and diffuser attachment like E.T. upon his arrival on earth and demurely asked, while holding it in front of his mouth like a microphone, 'What is this?'

"That's for Arielle to dry her hair," Chloe explained.

"Her hair doesn't dry on its own?"

"Well, no, it does, I guess. This just speeds up the process."

This explanation was met by a blank stare.

"You know, like making tea is faster if you use the electric kettle rather than the stove," she said.

An exaggerated nod of his head and symmetrical raise of his eyebrows tells her that he didn't really understand the point of this ominous contraption but has decided this hair-drying microphone might not be worth this much thinking.

"The other boys looked at it," Chloe said, "and as Mohammed held it in front of his face, I turned it on, and they all jumped back and then started laughing and took turns pointing it toward each other like a squirt gun."

Chloe's friend Monica was also there and suggested that they look at *Wet Hot American Summer,* which was among the DVDs in the house. They settle in to watch, with the three boys crushed closely together on the two kitchen chairs.

One scene is set at a typical New England summer camp. Tesh turns to Monica and asks, "Is this like an orphanage or something?"

"No, it's camp," Monica says, confused.

"What's camp? It looks like an orphanage."

"Yeah, I guess it does, sort of."

Solomon turns to Chloe and asks more quietly, "What is camp?" a lilting emphasis on camp.

She tries to explain summer camp in a way that makes it sound as unspoiled as possible. "It's a place like school where parents send their kids during the summer so they don't have to take care of them when they are not in school. It's like school, but you sleep there and it's fun."

Chloe went to camp once and left early. She hated it.

"I left them in peace to watch the movie," she remembers, "and curled up on the couch with my stolen Ethiopian Airlines blanket and *Of Mice and Men,* Mekonnen's and my next book. It began to rain again, as it has done every night these past weeks, despite every Ethiopian's assurance that this rain is extremely irregular for November and December, the Ethiopian summer months.

"They treat rain like corrosive acid rather than water," she said. "But I don't mind the rain. For me it's really just the mud that is tough. My shoes end up weighing more than I do at the end of a wet day. I am happy to hear the rain on the corrugated roofs. . . . As long as I am inside and the electricity stays on."

RICK TIMED ONE OF HIS REGULAR VISITS to New York to coincide with a benefit for FOCOS, Dr. Boachie's charity, and he took Zewdie with him as a flesh-and-blood example of what Dr. Boachie does with the contributions he receives. Then Zewdie traveled across the country with Rick and was particularly impressed with the Stanford University campus—suggesting that the standard of beauty and fine design may be universal—and stopped again in New York on his way home.

Rick had long wanted to meet Alan Alda. (He's such a great fan of *M*A*S*H* that he's memorized swaths of dialogue from the program.) Alan is a friend, so I arranged a dinner in New

York with him and some others I thought Rick and Zewdie would like.

Back in Addis about a month later, Zewdie, who had once planned to become an Orthodox priest, went with Rick to the mission on clinic day, where he started talking with an American Catholic priest visiting from New York City. Rick couldn't wait to send me an e-mail about the encounter.

> *Funny story: yesterday I was seeing patients and Zewdie was telling the priest that he was just in NYC as well, that he spoke at Cipriani's, he went to the top of the Empire State Building and had dinner with some actors. "I had dinner with Candice Bergen and Alan Alda," he told him. The priest looked at him like he was nuts.*
>
> *Later on, the priest and I were talking, and he told me what Zewdie had said. "It seemed too amazing," he said, "but the boy seemed so sincere and honest." I immediately opened up my computer and showed him a photo of Zewdie sitting on the couch with Alan and Candy, and the priest just smiled and shook his head.*

When Rick was in New York with Dr. Boachie, they talked about various patients, and Danny, the boy I had found on the street in Addis, was among them. The x-rays of his back showed that his deformity was unusually severe, especially considering how young he was, so he was chosen to be in the next group Rick was sending to Ghana. I suspected that another reason was that Danny has a way of charming the world, but Dr. Boachie described Danny as a ticking time bomb that might end in disaster if he wasn't cared for quickly. What he meant was that at his age, Danny could suffer a complete collapse of his spinal column that would cause paralysis and slow suffocation.

In November 2008, eleven months after our encounter on Arat Kilo, Danny and ten other Ethiopian boys and girls set out for their first airplane journey (having just taken their very first ride on an escalator as well) and headed for Ghana, where Dr. Boachie and his team would operate on their deformed backs. It was the beginning of a journey that could change their lives—if, as my mother used to say, all went well.

In a Thanksgiving e-mail, Rick reported on his latest group of spine patients:

> *Dr. Boachie and the entire FOCOS team*
> *could have been eating turkey with their families*
> *today, but rather traveled thousands of miles on*
> *their own dime and spent all day in the operating*
> *room in Accra operating on Danny. The surgery*
> *took so long that they had to postpone two of our*
> *other kids.*

Danny's surgery involved the removal of several fused vertebrae in a maneuver that few doctors know how to perform, as well as the implantation of two rods with titanium screws. He was on the operating table for eight and a half hours. Dr. Michael Mendelow, who had come from Detroit along with his own highly trained nurse, came into the OR for the final stage of the operation and saw that the monitors were indicating that Danny's spinal cord was not tolerating the closure of the wound.

Dr. Mendelow decided to insert a cross-link in his back, a brace under the skin that would protect the spinal cord. Without that maneuver, he said, Danny could very likely have become paralyzed. That gave me chills.

Dr. Boachie says that Danny's operation is the one he most hates to perform because of the dangers it presents to the spinal cord. Fortunately the FOCOS team had the equipment necessary to do what was needed.

I decided to stop in Ghana on my way to Ethiopia in December so I could see "my" little boy, and I arrived a few days after the surgery. The hospital was hot and not particularly clean, and Danny was lying on his cot like a sick puppy, all the oomph drained out of him. In the heat and humidity, Danny was wearing Spider Man flannel pajamas. His pink (!) Crocs were stowed under his bed. Berhanu, who goes to Ghana with each group of patients, was sitting with him.

Danny remembered me from the day I found him in the street, or at least he said he did. I'm still not sure whether he was just being polite—he has extraordinary social skills—or whether he really knew me. He just looked up at me with his big, sad eyes. It took the doctors a day or two to realize that he had been laid low by malaria, which happens to many of the children when they are given blood transfusions during surgery.

His neck and his back were hurting; he gamely agreed to walk a little—he was the first in the group to be up and around—but he was awfully weak. He seemed so miserable that I began to wonder if he wished I'd left him in the street. Fortunately, the malaria medication worked quickly, but it had been a real setback.

He liked the counting book I'd brought him because he's crazy about numbers, but he really sparked to the ballpoint pen that looked like a shark with toothy jaws that opened and lit up. He was devastated when it disappeared in the hospital—for a boy who'd never owned anything this had become a treasured possession—and I promised I'd look for another when I returned to the States. (Luckily I had my sales receipt and through the magic of the Internet and e-mail was able to find Laura Samuels at Hudson News, who donated a new one.)

Just before I left Ghana for Addis, I was able to visit Danny once again in the hospital. As he lay there, still a little achy from the malaria, I ran my finger along his cheek. "I love you," I told him.

Then it suddenly occurred to me to ask Berhanu if Danny knew what "love" is. He said he didn't.

By the time Danny returned to Addis on New Year's Day, 2009, Rick had already been to Rwanda and back and had offered to work in Zimbabwe when a cholera epidemic struck there.

"Nobody's had more experience with cholera than I've had," he said.

I breathed a sigh of relief when no one took him up on his offer. Rick was less happy. He's irrepressible in his search for people to make better.

A friend in Ethiopia once told him that expatriates fall under one of the 3Ms: missionaries, mercenaries, and misfits.

"Since I am neither of the first two," he said, "I suppose that makes me a misfit."

If so, he's a misfit who is trying to persuade others to follow in his unconventional footsteps. Whatever sacrifices he has made in the way of building his own financial security, whatever ease and luxuries he has forsworn, he'd do it all over again.

He constantly urges young people, as he did at a recent graduation, to look for something that really interests them, to have a sense of "wow, I get to go to work today." He tells them to seek out meaning, not money. He tells students to take time off to see the world.

"Let me tell you," he says, "at my age, *nobody*, really nobody, says, 'Wow, I'm really happy that I went straight from college to law school.'"

In 2008, Rick was awarded a mastership by the American College of Physicians, the professional organization of internists in the United States, which made him one of an elite "group of highly distinguished physicians . . . who have achieved recognition in medicine by exhibiting preeminence in practice or medical research, holding positions of high honor, or making significant contributions to medical science or the art of medicine."

The citation said those receiving a mastership are selected because of "personal character, and must be highly accomplished individuals . . . distinguished by the excellence and significance of his or her contributions to the field of medicine."

Rick was cited for initiatives combining medical acumen, savvy about the medical care environments that are in play, tenacious advocacy on behalf of disenfranchised and very ill patients without medical care and, not least of all, his "unconditional love" for fellow human beings.

The next year the same organization awarded him the prestigious Rosenthal Award, given to "the physician-scientist, clinician, or scientific group whose recent innovative work is making a notable contribution to improve clinical care in the field of internal medicine."

Not bad for a guy who's been in Ethiopia for two decades!

Rick prefers to understate his accomplishments.

"I've taken to calling myself a travel agent," he says. "My

goal? Mostly, it's to use the world's medical resources simply to help people continue their present journey on this planet. I perceive my role here as assisting people at the margins whom nobody else will help.

"I'm a believer in the Woody Allen school of thought: showing up is a lot of the job. At the end of the day what keeps me going is my reward in knowing that a few more people may be alive because I went to work that day."

12

MY LUCKY DAY

H ERE IS DANNY, SINGING IN THE bathtub and looking out the window at Central Park. It is one year and two months since I found him, a homeless and crippled waif, beseeching passersby for coins that might add up to a meager dinner.

"You are my sunshine," he pipes as he spreads his right arm out wide. "You are my sunshine," now out to the left. "You make me happy, when skies are gra-a-a-ay," now both arms, as if playing to the audience like a contestant on *American Idol* but looking more like Al Jolson without the white gloves.

"You Are My Sunshine" is a song Rick uses to awaken the kids at home, and now Danny is performing, all agiggle, his two missing front teeth not inhibiting him at all.

Sometimes he changes the words to "You are my shoeshine," an ode to one of the boys in the Hodes house who used to shine

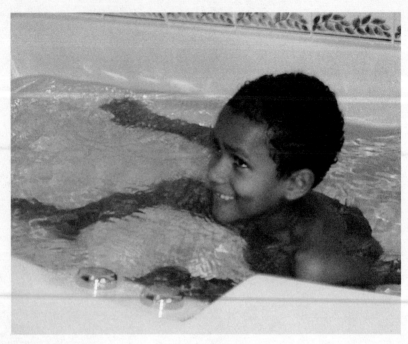

You are my sunshine.

shoes but could no longer ply his trade after his back surgery. "You are my shoeshine, Yilak," he shouts, a mischievous gleam in his eye.

As I watch this performance, I can still see the beautiful but dirty and destitute little ragamuffin in the middle of the street, even though before me now is this new (and real) vision of a joyous kid who loves to scrub and splash and sing. There is no sound more delicious than his laughter ringing out through the entire apartment. His gleeful shouts are changing my life too.

He is here on a visit. Rick was coming to the States, and I suggested that since Danny couldn't go to school until his back healed, he might benefit from a bit of time in New York to learn English. To say nothing about what it would do for me.

So on a Sunday afternoon my husband, Don, and I met Rick and his little sidekick at the airport. As they emerged from immigration, we waved our arms and shouted, "Danny, Danny!" to get his attention and to make him feel welcome in this strange new world. He was still suffering the aftereffects of air sickness, but he flashed a big smile and came right over with his hand extended in a manly greeting. We let Rick walk ahead while Don and I each took one of Danny's hands. It didn't take him long to ask me if I had found another shark pen.

Danny came home with us while Rick, wearing his customary hand-crocheted red-and-yellow-and-blue-striped Ethiopian beanie (that always makes me think of Puck in *A Midsummer Night's Dream*), made his way to the West Side YMCA, his home away from home. His room is like a monk's cell, but the Y is inexpensive and well located, and it has a swimming pool.

Before they arrived I had tried to find an Amharic translator to make Danny feel more comfortable, but from the first day he had no problem making himself understood. Anything would do for lunch and dinner—as long as it's meat for this little refugee from a vegetarian household. For breakfast it was warm milk with three sugars and four slices of whole wheat toast. His face grew worried one morning when he noticed that we were getting to the end of the loaf; his previous experiences of running out of food had not been good ones. I quickly showed him the fresh new package of bread and got a relieved smile.

He had no trouble eating four lamb chops (his favorite) at one sitting and—for a forty-pound skinny kid—he downed an astonishing amount of hamburgers, meatballs, ribs, steak, and pasta. One day, while our housekeeper, Charlette, was cooking, he wandered into the kitchen to ask what she was making.

"Chips," she replied, his name for the French fries he adores. He gave her a big hug, and she was happy for the rest of the week.

He turned out to be my kind of kid. He discovered he likes ice cream (vanilla), sleeps long and late, as I do, and can read anything, whether in a book or on a street sign. I still don't know how, during his first days in New York, he was able to read "NYPD" as New York Police Department. When the wind blew too hard, he ran into a vestibule to warm up, and with his teeth chattering, informed me with great seriousness that "Ethiopia is not too hot, not too cold."

As we walked along, to the park or to the grocery, he volunteered that he's a fan of Chris Brown, Eminem, and 50 Cent (so we're not in tune about everything). MTV is supposed to be off-limits in the Hodes house, but the boys watch it a lot when Rick isn't looking. In America, Danny seemed to prefer *Tom and Jerry* (he favors Jerry, who is small and feisty and plays tricks on Tom), and he became transfixed by video games that he plays with a lot of body English, practically dancing while he manipulates the controller of GameCube.

It soon became very difficult to pry him away from that mesmerizing contraption, but we eventually walked over to the Museum of Natural History. He could read the names of all the animals and loved the IMAX dinosaurs, but he blew my mind when he saw a picture of a human skeleton. He looked up at me and in the most matter-of-fact manner said, "Is that Lucy?" I asked if he had seen Lucy, the earliest humanlike skeleton that was unearthed in Ethiopia, in the Addis museum.

"We don't have museums in Ethiopia," he said incorrectly.

The next day there was a photograph of the actual Lucy skeleton in the newspaper and I said, "Danny, who's that?"

"Lucy," he replied, as if everybody would know that. Wow. These Ethiopians sure know their ancestors.

This was when I discovered that this isn't just a soul. Danny has one very sharp mind.

And that was only the beginning. One day while he was in the bathtub, he looked up at me and Charlette, whom he had heard calling me "Madame," and, taking a page from *The Cat in the Hat* where he was introduced to Thing 1 and Thing 2, said, "You're Madame 1, and you're Madame 2."

I was knocked out by his ability to transfer the metaphor in a new language. As he met our friends, they were also astonished by his English vocabulary and his amazing ease as he adjusted to new people and new situations. He remembers everything he's ever seen or heard. Maybe he "inherited" that talent from Rick.

At breakfast one morning, Danny informed us that Barack Obama is America's forty-fourth president.

"How did you know that," we asked.

"When I was in Ghana, it was on a T-shirt, Obama and 44," he explained.

Okay, good enough. But then he told us Bush was forty-three. And before that?

"Clinton, forty-two," he responded immediately.

And before that?

"Bush, forty-one."

And before that?

Reagan, he informed us, was the fortieth president. Wow again.

Danny went off to spend the weekend with our two grandsons, whose house is a toyland of robots, video games, LEGOs—more of everything, I guessed, than exists in all of Ethiopia. When we took him away from the boys to another house for dinner, he sat in a heartbreaking funk for an hour until he started playing with a new boy he'd been brought there to meet. And he brightened considerably when the steak was served.

"This is good," the young food critic remarked.

In the basement of our apartment building, we found a game room I'd forgotten was there because I had no children—until now. Danny leapt on the foosball (eat your heart out, Mesfin!) and the Ping-Pong table and the hobbyhorse with a mane of real hair. One night, as I was putting him to bed in his fresh snowflake-patterned pajamas (he calls them *b-jamas*), he said, "I don't want to go back to Ethiopia."

My heart leapt and sank at the same time.

Danny wasn't with us a week when our rollicking high spirits were shattered by a thunderbolt. My husband was diagnosed with pancreatic cancer that would require immediate hospitalization and surgery. Clearly this wasn't the best time for Danny to be visiting us—it was in fact impossible—so I asked Rick what he thought of asking Nancy Larson, his old buddy from the Goma refugee camp, to take the boy for a month. She has a daughter, Lydia, who is just a little younger than Danny. I knew Nancy only from a long telephone conversation in which we discussed her work with Rick and the story of how Taka, the Rwandan refugee child who was saved from certain death after he was beaten with a machete, came into her life when he was brought back to their encampment after surgery in that Israeli field hospital.

Asking her to take Danny for a month was a pretty nervy thing to do, but I wasn't surprised when she agreed immediately. Nancy is what we used to call the salt of the earth. She is kind and giving and loves to laugh.

Nancy came to our New York apartment so she and Danny could get to know each other before she took him to Minneapolis. When they left after a few days, an uncomfortable silence fell over our household, and Danny's piping voice enlivened the precincts of Maple Grove, Minnesota, the Larsons' neighborhood. He and the Larson daughter, Lydia, have become devoted sister and brother, and I worry not at all that she's taught him all sorts of girlie games, including things like how to give tea parties. He was also taken to the family farm, where he got to ride on a huge tractor and see the farm animals and play with the twenty-four cousins who'd come for Easter weekend. He went fishing on Lake Minnetonka, one of Minnesota's ten thousand lakes. Danny will come back, we told ourselves, when Don is better. But I missed him terribly.

Once Don was released from the hospital, all of the Larsons came east to bring Danny to our house in the country, where Danny proceeded to captivate everybody in town. His English had improved 1,000 percent. He understands everything and can say anything—and often does, at length. One of my nephews urged me to describe him as voluble, but that's an understatement. He never tires of relating in excruciating detail the plots of movies; he reads with great fluency; he loves numbers and likes to count everything and anything; he's a whiz at the computer. The town librarian, mother of one girl, went off on excursions of imagination at the thought of adopting him.

Danny swallowed books whole and loved to have me read to him, but he also loved to read to me, and he would sometimes sing the words in his lovely boy soprano. At the end of his song, the ham in him takes over, and he becomes a rock star after a performance.

"Thank you, thank you very much," he says, clutching his hands to his heart. "Thank you. *Amasegenalow*. Thank you."

Then like a rock star, pointing at one person in his imaginary audience—"you, over there"—he would start again, addressing the phantom with another heartfelt "thank you, thank you."

And what are the chances that I'd find two Ethiopian boys not five minutes from our house, brothers adopted by a wonderful couple who live literally down the street? I had my first experience with playdates. Whenever he was invited over to Habtamu and Lire's house, his face lit up in a huge smile.

"Today?" he would ask eagerly. "When do we go?"

These kids play an enthusiastic and rather undisciplined soccer game, and Danny is always chosen first for any team. He seems to know instinctively that if he passes the ball, he will be a popular team player—his social skills come naturally—but he also dribbles down the field and scores more often than anybody. With each successful goal, he crosses the field in an exuberant dash, smiling from ear to ear, running with his arms out in a spread-eagle victory lap—sometimes known as the airplane—like a miniature David Beckham, and then pumping his fists vigorously.

At home Danny delighted in scaring the living daylights out of me, hiding behind doors and under beds at every opportunity and then jumping out at me with a devilish shriek and an impish smile that dissolved me into a quivering puddle of affection. He informed me that in Ethiopia, you can only scare somebody once. Here, with me, it worked every time.

He was thrilled with his new bike and his Spider Man helmet, which he insisted on wearing backward. He became entranced with a boy doll a friend brought him that translates English to

Spanish, and one day I found him opening the back where a seam covered the internal battery.

"Shh," he told me when I interrupted his concentration, "I'm operating on his back."

After he finished "sewing up" the doll, he said to him, "Now you cannot eat for two days. I couldn't eat for two days after I had surgery." He says he wants to be a back surgeon when he grows up. I think he can be anything he wants.

"It was my lucky day when I met you," I told Danny one evening.

"No," he replied, "it was *my* lucky day."

Once word got out among our friends that Danny was with us, our social life expanded exponentially and we were on everybody's A-list. Danny's dance card was full for the Memorial Day weekend. One friend opened her grandchildren's game room to him where he had access to every kind of video game. He—and therefore, we—were invited to lunch at another house on both Saturday and Sunday, where he was asked to help build a tree house. Here he found a big and boisterous family, where the mother thought Danny was the cat's pajamas and wanted him to stay with them for the entire summer. Regrettably, Rick thought it would be too hard on him to return to Ethiopia after three months with an American family that has everything.

But there seems to be no situation he can't deal with, no child—or adult—he cannot relate to. He prattles on and on and plays with words. Joan Ganz Cooney, the founder of Sesame Street, declared that Danny is the single smartest child she's ever met in her life. She said she would bet he has an IQ of 150—an estimate she shortly revised to 180 as she got to know him better. And she knows whereof she speaks. Her concern is that he get the best possible education available in the world because she feels his potential is enormous. Rick—and I—will see to that.

Rick had gone back to Addis and returned to the States, stopping in New York City on his way to somewhere else. The three of us had dinner, and Rick told Danny what I had been dreading all along, that he'd be taking him back to Addis in about ten days; the visit was over.

Danny, it turned out, seemed far more ready to accept this than I was, and he started looking forward to eating some of his favorite Ethiopian dishes. He was worried about his bicycle. He wanted to take it with him on the plane. I explained that Rick thinks it is too dangerous to ride bikes in Addis but that I would keep it here for him to ride next summer.

But while I had him, each night, Danny would cuddle into my arms and, with a smile that was impossible to refuse (even if I'd wanted to), ask me to take turns reading with him. I'd read the page on the left and he the right. His favorite bedtime story was *The Trumpet of the Swan,* and he loved to mimic me as I mimicked the deep voice of the self-important father swan. "Here I glide, swanlike . . . while earth is bathed in wonder and beauty . . . while eggs hatch, while young swans come into existence. . . . I glide, I glide swanlike."

Danny's laughter is uncontained when he reads the swan's mate reply. "Of course you glide like a swan. . . . How else could you glide? You couldn't glide like a moose, could you?"

Every now and then Danny would open up about that part of his life that he'd been trying so hard to shut out. He is officially a ward of the Mother Teresa Mission, but he told me he remembers his mother; he just doesn't know where she is. At night, he says they used to sleep huddled together, his mother and two younger brothers, in the vestibule of a store on Bole Road. They had to get up early before the pedestrians shooed them away. By day, after washing up from a Highland Water bottle, they made Bole Road their turf, where they scrounged for money with their hands out.

Danny said he would get 10 birr to every 5 his mother took in, probably because his back was so seriously deformed that passersby were more generous with him. He says he thinks his back had started to hump out when he was about three, and as he grew, his back got "bigger," as he puts it. The reason he begged, he said, was that his mother was hungry. He told me the police took away a three-year-old brother he adored because his mother couldn't care for him. A baby brother remained with his mother, probably because he was still being breast-fed, and he says he doesn't know where they are now. Nor does he know the whereabouts of several older brothers, all but one of them sons of different fathers.

With all that, he has good memories of his mother. He smiles most sweetly when he talks about her and says he'd be happy to see her again. His mother taught him many things, he says. It was she who told him about Lucy, known as Dinkenesh (meaning "you are beautiful or you are wonderful"), the 3.2-million-year-old hominid skeleton that was found in the Afar Depression of Ethiopia. He says she also taught him never to smoke, and she taught him the names of many countries in the world—which has made him very good at Geography, a game we play in the car to pass the time. Imagine how I felt when he told me that his mom had told him it would be best for him if he could get to America.

But the stepfather was another story. One evening, as he was having his nightly portion of vanilla ice cream, Danny told me his stepfather could be violent and each night took the money he had collected and used it to buy arak and beer. He would beat the boy—and sometimes brutally beat Danny's mother—with a *same,* a sort of leaf apparently similar to a stinging nettle that hurts for an hour after it hits the skin. Well, nobody messes with Danny, who had a healthy sense of his own value now that he was collecting twice as much on the street as his mother. He got angry—and he got even; his stepfather had beaten him for the last time. One day, while the family was working the precincts of Bole Road and not long after his little brother was taken away, Danny took his meager stash of birr and ran away to Arat Kilo, the main thoroughfare where I found him that January day.

Well, he didn't exactly run away. He took a taxi! It was one of those diesel blue and white jobs that look to be fifty years old and spew black smoke into the street and onto the passengers they carry. Danny said he recognized a man in the passenger seat of this particular taxi and jumped in. On arriving at Arat Kilo, he started handing the fare to the driver, but the man told him to keep his money.

So began the saga of Danny making his way in the world on his own. Age: six or seven.

His heartrendingly deformed back caused passersby to be relatively generous to him. He didn't need much to get along. With 2 birr (about 20 cents), he happily told me, he could have a dinner of *miser wat* (lentil stew) with *ingera*; with 3 birr he could get *bayenet* with *gomen* (a kind of macaroni with vegetable sauce and salad). One birr would get him tea and biscuits.

But how did he feel when he was all alone on the street away from his mother and brother? Was he frightened or lonely? Not at all, he said. He could get money to eat, and anyway he had two older friends, Abel and Andahem, who knew their way around. He could indulge his passion for video games. If he lost, he paid. If he won, his opponent paid for the next round.

He liked being on his own with no one to tell him what to do, and to this day he bristles when he is asked to do anything he'd rather not. When I asked if he ever went to school before he ended up at Rick's, he said, "No. No money."

There are certain mysteries that remain about Danny. He has secrets, he says. "It's complicated." If you make the mistake of going too far and asking too many questions about his past, Danny stops abruptly. "The End," he says. "The movie is over."

But there were occasional insights unintentionally offered. As we watched the movie *The Black Stallion,* in which a boy survives a shipwreck and is left alone, I remarked that this was scary.

"Not scary," Danny replied, "sad, but not scary. As long as he can get food to eat and something to drink, he'll be all right."

It turns out that Danny's sojourn on Arat Kilo may have been far shorter than I at first thought. He thinks he had been there only three or four days when Chloe and I happened along.

In June, Danny returned to Addis with Rick, and our house again fell silent. It seemed empty. I heard from friends in Addis that Danny was crying at night, that he said this was the hour I used to read to him. That hurt. I immediately started lobbying Rick to see if he wanted to come back. The truth is that I became terrifically preoccupied with him—perhaps obsessed is the proper word—and finally asked Rick to bring him when he returned at the beginning of July. We couldn't stand not having him here. Typically, Rick didn't answer for a long time, and I became—not to put too fine a point on it—pretty annoying as I harassed him by e-mail for an answer.

At last Rick wrote that he had offered Danny a choice: he could stay in Addis and go to summer school; he could return with him to the States for a two-week visit; or he could come to our house for the entire summer. Guess what he chose?

Wrong! He chose to stay in Addis. I suppose home is home. But at this point, I told Rick, I was a little insulted. So I telephoned Danny and asked why he didn't want to come. He said he did. My spirits soared.

When he arrived, we picked up where we left off, except that we enrolled Danny in a day camp. Each morning when he got to camp, both the counselors and the kids seemed excited to see him. They waved and shouted, "Hey, Danny." He'd return the greeting or—always with a sweet smile—yell "loser" to taunt some counselor who had led a losing team the day before. He was supposed to stay each day until 1:00 P.M. He chose to stay until three so he could play chess!

We got word that Danny scored 97 percent in his first-grade placement exam in Addis. He had the highest grade, so the school asked that he come back to take the third-grade entry exam. I decided to teach him multiplication so he'd be ready, but he already knew it. I asked him how he'd learned it, and he informed me that a wizard had come by and implanted it in his brain. We need the wizard back to do fractions.

By this time, Don's condition was worsening. Thankfully, he was not in pain, but he got thinner and thinner and said he couldn't understand why. He saw no relation between his weight loss and his illness. He'd get himself up each day and often went out looking for the new car he planned to buy next year when his current auto lease ran out. He kidded around with Danny.

"Whadda boy!" he would say, and Danny beamed back happily.

It didn't take us long to realize that we could never let Danny go after the summer. There was no way we could officially adopt him because Ethiopian law requires that the parent be no more than forty years older than the child. Frankly, both Don and I were decades beyond the age limit, and there appeared to be no provision for adoption by grandparents. But we could give him, as I like to say, room, board, and love.

This was totally uncharacteristic for me. When I was single, and admittedly that was for quite a long time, I wouldn't even take on the responsibility of a plant because it would have to be watered. Now I was ready to take on a child. I realized I was living my life totally backward, and I was defying my biological clock: graduation from college, a career, a late marriage, semi-retirement, and finally—motherhood. Since I was no longer working twenty-hour days I had, for the first time in my life, time to be a mother. But only a woman who never had a child would be foolhardy enough to take on such a daunting task, particularly at my age.

Danny was a ward of Mother Teresa's, but Rick had been given full authority to make decisions about his health and his education. Danny was already showing great potential academically, so Rick agreed to allow us to find a school for him in New York. It was August. Friends asked where I was going to send him. "Whatever school answers the phone," I would reply.

As it turned out, four of the city's best private schools answered the phone. One day as we were leaving for a school interview, Danny looked up at my hair, which was still wet from my morning shower; it is always very curly and, to be honest, totally impossible in the summer months.

"Are you going that way?" he asked. "In Ethiopia, you know, women do wonderful things with their hair." What could I say?

Danny was accepted at all of the schools that interviewed him. One admissions officer said, "I could have spent the whole day with him."

We chose the one closest to home so his pals would be in the neighborhood. He's in second grade. He zooms to school on a scooter. I try to keep up, an excellent form of exercise for the day.

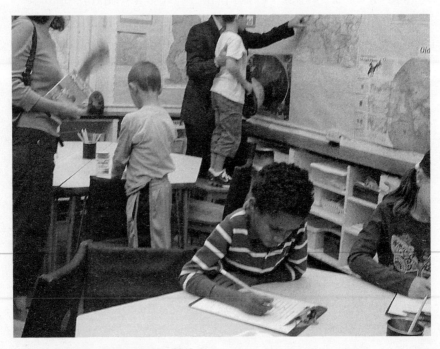

Danny's first day of school in New York City.

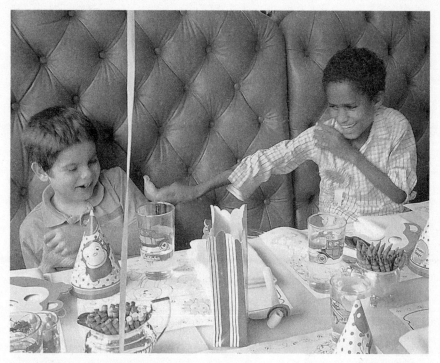

Danny, eight, at his very first birthday party.

His new student visa allows him to stay in the United States as long as he goes to school.

Don never got to see Danny start school. He took a last deep breath on August 19 as I sat holding his hand.

Rick had told me I'd saved Danny's life. Now he was saving mine.

Danny left me with little time to dwell on the upheaval in my life. I had to get up uncharacteristically early in the morning to coax him out of bed and walk him to school, and I had to devote myself to his well-being, not my own. As we were walking home from school one day, Danny looked up at me and said, "Instead of a dog, could we get a fish?" A *dog,* I thought. I had

257

given my life over to a child; I couldn't even contemplate having a dog. Well, I can tell you, you never saw anybody buy a fish so quickly. Danny named the goldfish Bob, after a dog they'd had at the house in Addis who had died. He now had a responsibility, to feed Bob.

One day he looked in the fish tank and said, "Bob looks lonely." I suggested that he might be better off here in our house than in the basement of the fish store. "Yes," Danny said, "but in the fish store he had friends." I understood that he was having trouble adjusting to a household with no kids after the many he lived with in Ethiopia.

After about a month in school, he asked if he could have a nanny like the other kids. Some of my friends had hired young men to take care of their boys and that seemed like a good idea for a child who had no father at home. So I found a "manny." His name is also Daniel. I asked Danny one Friday if he would mind if Daniel took him to his piano lesson because I was busy. "Why not," he replied. "He's my best friend!"

Soon I enrolled Danny in a soccer program. On his first day there, one of the boys looked at him and said, "Who the heck are you?"

"I'm the new boy," Danny replied. He then proceeded to make five goals himself so everybody knew who the heck he is. His soccer coach at school has given him a nickname: Prodigy.

Oh no, now I'm a soccer mom!

The first big snowfall of the year was also Danny's first look at heavy snow, requiring a search for a good hill. We had no sled and the stores were sold out, but I figured somebody would lend us one for a few minutes.

As we surveyed the scene, he clearly had his doubts, but

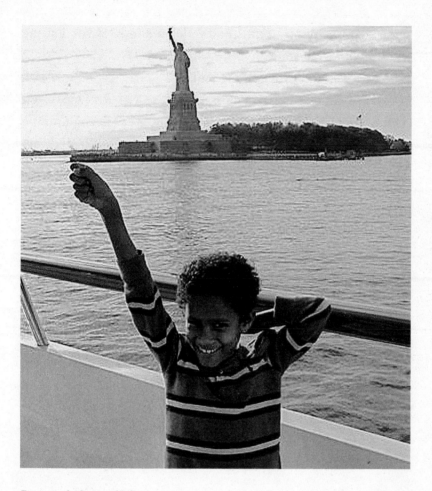

Danny at the Statue of Liberty.

when a nice guy allowed us to use his sled (devoid of any steering mechanism), Danny agreed to give it a try—provided I go with him. As I calculate it, I hadn't been on a sled for some fifty years. But why not?

We piled on and immediately went off course and onto the bumpy side of the hill.

"That was totally not good," Danny declared. "Let's try

again." This time we went straight down and he arrived at the bottom with a big smile.

"That was totally good," he said.

Danny came with me to a memorial service for Don, a celebration of his extraordinary life as a pioneer of television in the twentieth century and a creator of *60 Minutes*. Don had always told us in the family never to be sad when he died.

"I've had the best life," he would say. "It has to end some time."

A couple of days after the memorial, Danny was having his nightly portion of ice cream, now a mix of vanilla and chocolate.

"What's your biggest wish in the whole world?" he asked me.

I said something about wanting him to be happy and then said, "What's your biggest wish?"

"My biggest, my most important wish in the whole world," he said, starting off slowly and pointing at the table, "is that Don would be right here and see me in my Spider Man Halloween costume and he would say, 'Whadda boy!'"

EPILOGUE

WHEN I ARRIVED IN ADDIS FOR the first time, it was 4:00 A.M. and I was more than ready to take to my bed after a twenty-two-hour flight. But there was a note under my door:

> *I'm picking up eight patients arriving at 9:00 A.M.*
> *at the airport from Gondar where they had surgery.*
> *Do you want to come?*

No, I did not want to come, but I couldn't afford to miss it. This would be my first meeting with Rick, whom I'd come halfway around the world to see.

"Seeing these people after surgery is like going to heaven," Rick exulted as he greeted them at Bole Airport. And in time I realized that in this single sentence was the key to Rick Hodes. If a diamond ring makes one person happy, and an ice cream cone another, helping people is what makes Rick positively ecstatic. There is something in the pleasure center of his brain that is turned on and brings him joy when he helps people. As I got to know him, one e-mail after another would end with "We're happy we can help him." And he means it.

So I returned to the question I'd asked at the beginning. What makes a Rick? I'm not the only person trying to find out. There are research institutes on two coasts with impressive boards of directors and staffed with serious scientists—one at Stanford and another in Stony Brook, Long Island (called the Institute for Research on Unlimited Love)—trying to discover the roots of altruism and compassion, and the means of fostering such behavior.

Numerous books and papers have been written, taking into account evolution, neurology, and even neuroeconomics, but the study of this phenomenon is still in a fairly primitive state.

It is too early, I am told, to discover where in the brain the joy of altruism may be seated, but there is no question that giving, in all its variations, provides pleasure. Experiments prove it. And this is true whether one does good for the right reasons or for the wrong ones. If one gives to enhance one's stature in the community, is that to be looked upon with cynicism? Even philanthropists of that sort get the feeling that scientists have unscientifically called the warm glow.

One thing the students of the phenomenon are learning is that even people who are self-absorbed and narcissistic can, through training, learn altruism. Believe me, if I could learn it, anyone can. And I have no doubt I learned it from Rick.

As for Rick, his life has now come full circle. Israel has announced that it is ready to take in more Ethiopian Jews and has asked Rick to open a clinic to process them. On Thanksgiving day in 2009, he wrote,

I'm in Gondar where we're reopening our clinic
here for well over five thousand people. Had the
first fifty-two families today, went fine. Now
I have four or five hours of data to analyze.

Rick then got word that the new clinic will not serve five thousand patients. The number had gone up to nine thousand. "I'll have a busy month coming up," Rick said. He sounded like he couldn't wait to take on more work.

Three Israeli parliamentarians came to visit him at the Gondar clinic at the end of November 2009. Among them was Professor Arieh Eldad, former chief of plastic surgery at Hadassah Hospital and former surgeon general of the Israeli Defense Forces. It was not his first visit to Ethiopia. He was the surgeon in the Israeli field hospital in Goma who took care of the little Rwandan boy who was smashed in the head with a machete, the boy who was adopted by the Larsons in Minnesota. Rick said, "he fondly remembered operating on Taka in Goma, Zaire, with a 'Japanese paper knife.'"

It's uncanny how these things keep happening to Rick. I told him that Walter Cronkite used to say there are only four hundred people in the world: "They do it with mirrors." Rick took a picture of the doctor to send to Taka. "Last time he saw me he was under anesthesia and I was wearing a mask," Dr. Eldad said.

In Addis this year, the Ethiopian government undertook an intensive scrutiny of Rick's work. "Met with them and summarized my work," he said. "They interviewed my staff without me. They interviewed my patients without me present. They looked intensely at the mission." In the end, the ministry of health gave him a superb evaluation and asked him to expand. That won't be easy. There's only one of him.

At the end of December 2009, Rick sent a brief update on his projects:

Yesterday was my last clinic day of the year. Got one new spine on Sat, two on Friday. I am excited to sit down and work on my statistics.

I have a great and active seven-year-old boy with Hodgkin's who is responding well to ABVD—one week after treatment #1, his mass has decreased about 10 percent.

I also decided to treat a twenty-one-year-old with T-cell lymphoblastic lymphoma. I did that a week ago, he improved a bit, then died two days later. I may have slightly hastened his death, but am happy that I was able to give him a shot at life.

One of my heart patients who had been to India stopped taking her meds a month ago (she was on blood thinners) and came into the mission, very sick. She died the next day. We all feel bad, but she was fully informed about the need to stay on meds for the rest of her life. "After that," I always say, "you don't need them."

I prob have ten patients, maybe even a dozen, with pure mitral stenosis, which can be ballooned open in Cochin for $1500 each. I am thinking about addressing this in the first half of 2010 if I can get the money together. It's painful to see them all, knowing that their time is slowly slipping away, when their valve area is down to 0.6 cm.

Two more kids with big lymphomas in Dire Dawa. The nuns called to ask if it would be possible to send them to me. ("Today," I replied.)

The Ghana gang is recovering well, last clinic visit may be on Monday, and they may be back on Wed.

So it goes. Stay warm.

Rick

Not long before this e-mail arrived, Danny and I were decorating a Christmas tree, his first—and mine, too.

"This is the best day of my life," he declared.

So it goes.

ACKNOWLEDGMENTS

THIS BOOK WOULD NOT EXIST without Jo Ann Silverstein, who returned from Ethiopia at the end of 2007 full of enthusiasm and excitement about a doctor she met doing good work in Ethiopia. She wondered if I knew anyone who might want to write about him. As if in involuntary response, my right hand went up, and so began this tale.

Chloe Malle, who accompanied me on my first trip to Addis, was a support then and became my boots on the ground when she decided to spend almost a year working with Rick as a volunteer.

Robert Fishman, my (thankfully) live-in nephew, who was my first reader. He offered insightful comments and guided me through recurring technological near-disasters.

Laura Yorke, my agent, who helped me navigate the publishing world in two days of whirlwind presentations that raised great interest in the book.

Henry Ferris, my editor, who loves a good story chronologically told. He was unusually welcoming when I arrived at William Morrow with my proposal and that, combined with the unbridled enthusiasm of Vice President Seale Ballenger, who was virtually jumping up and down with passion for the project when we first met, made this publishing house irresistible.

Nancy Larson, who, at a critical moment in my life, filled in for me with generosity and love.

Amir Shaviv, my rabbi at the American Jewish Joint Distribution Committee (JDC), helped me navigate some surprisingly thorny issues raised in that organization by the idea of my writing this book, and Slava Mitsel, who guided me through the JDC's extensive archive of photos from Operation Solomon and the refugee camps.

And, most of all, Rick Hodes, who throughout this entire process generously shared with me his recollections and his humor and who enriched my life by teaching me, through his example, the meaning of compassion. His wholehearted commitment was contagious, and from that I now have the joy and pleasure of a little boy whose life he saved.

Last, but certainly not least, my husband, Don Hewitt, who, no matter how sick he became, remained my cheerleader and provided unfailing support, and whose spirit never wavered in his devotion to me, to this story, and to Danny. He made it all possible.

If you would like to help fund lifesaving surgeries for Dr. Hodes's patients, tax-exempt contributions can be sent to him through the American Jewish Joint Distribution Committee (JDC), P.O. Box 530, 132 East 43rd Street, New York, NY 10017. The JDC passes 100 percent of all money earmarked for Rick Hodes directly to him without deducting any administrative costs.

Dr. Boachie, the spine surgeon, receives contributions through the Foundation for Orthopedics and Complex Spine (FOCOS), P.O. Box 665, Lenox Hill Station, New York, NY 10021.